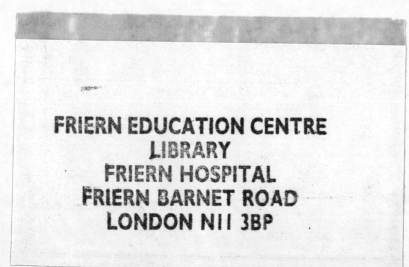
i

For Polly, Ben and Kerry

For Churchill Livingstone
Publisher: Mary Law
Project Editor: Dinah Thom
Editorial Co-ordination: Editorial Resources Unit
  Copy Editor: Joanna Smith
Production Controller: Nancy Henry
Design: Design Resources Unit
Sales Promotion Executive: Hilary Brown

The Nursing Process in Psychiatry

Martin F. Ward

RMN DN(Lond) CertEd(Leeds) RNT NEBSSDip
Lecturer in Mental Health Nursing Studies
Norfolk College of Nursing and Midwifery ·
Hellesdon Hospital, Norwich

SECOND EDITION

CHURCHILL LIVINGSTONE
EDINBURGH LONDON MADRID MELBOURNE NEW YORK AND TOKYO 1992

CHURCHILL LIVINGSTONE
Medical Division of Longman Group UK Limited

Distributed in the United States of America by Churchill
Livingstone Inc., 650 Avenue of the Americas, New York,
N.Y. 10011, and by associated companies, branches and
representatives throughout the world.

First edition 1985
Second edition 1992

ISBN 0-443-04225-X

British Library Cataloguing in Publication Data
A catalogue record for this book is available from the British
Library

Library of Congress Cataloging in Publication Data
Ward, Martin F.
   The nursing process in psychiatry/Martin F. Ward. -- 2nd ed.
      p.   cm.
   Includes bibliographical references and index.
   ISBN 0-443-04225-X
   1. psychiatric nursing.   I. Title.
   [DNLM: 1. Nursing Process.   2. Psychiatric Nursing--methods.   WY
160 W261n]
RC400.W34   1992
610.73'68--dc20
DNLM/DLC
for Library of Congress   91-29752

Produced by Longman Singapore Publishers (Pte) Ltd.
Printed in Singapore

Preface to second edition

Much has happened in the world since the first edition of this book was published in 1985. Significantly, the whole approach to the development and consolidation of contemporary psychiatric nursing practice has swung very much in favour of the nurses themselves. Legislation, education and aspiration have all conspired to make this a very exciting time for nurses in the many clinical specialisms of psychiatry. One thing that has not altered is the nurse's need for knowledge and consequently the necessity for nursing authors to provide up-to-date information about everything from philosophical baselines to advanced care strategies. Today, nurses are expected to manage their own budgets, coordinate care teams, function within complicated management structures, use modern personal and computerised technology and still deliver a quality of care that is consistent with the highest standards of nursing intervention. This new edition has taken much from the original book and enhanced it with new ideas and technology in an attempt to help the nurse achieve the last of these priorities.

The basic approach to the nursing process remains unchanged but I have produced new care plans which hopefully will enable the reader more fully to appreciate their use. A new chapter looks at objective setting, still one of the main difficulties experienced by nurses using the process, whilst another chapter considers the relationship between the nursing process and effective patient–nurse communication. The community chapter has been placed in a more appropriate part of the book and now contains a care study to illustrate the use of the process in this area.

One of the most important issues being addressed by nurses is the rights and dignity of the patients with whom they work. The collaboration between patients and nurses is at the heart of an effective nursing process, yet in psychiatry this may not always easily be achieved. I have tried to bring this problem into focus as much as possible throughout the text, though the reader may disagree with some of my views on the way this should be approached. However, this should not obscure the main argument, that patients have the right both to be involved, and to opt out of being involved, in decisions which affect their care. The nursing process remains the single tool available to nurses to enable this activity to take place without the patient being disadvantaged by whichever decision he/she makes.

Once again, although I have made alterations to suit the text much of the material in this edition reflects the work of the psychiatric care teams within the Norwich Health Authority. I am grateful to them for their commitment to the process and their continuing desire to improve upon its effectiveness.

Finally, I apologise in advance to those readers who expect authors to solve the problem of patient/nurse gender within a text without forever using him/her. I have been unable to assign a particular gender to either group, except where discussing individual cases. In the main, however, I have identified the patient as male and the nurse as female.

Norwich, 1992   M.F.W.

Preface to first edition

This book has been written in an attempt to provide practising psychiatric nurses with a guide to the implementation of the nursing process in their own discipline. Surprisingly enough, there are very few texts available to United Kingdom nurses which relate the process to the very special needs and peculiarities of psychiatry. Yet despite comments made in much of the nursing press, the process is definitely here to stay. It is not just another transitory system adopted by the nursing intelligentsia, but a very real and practical philosophy designed to improve the effectiveness of the care that patients receive. Almost half of the current syllabus used to train the new generation of psychiatric nurses uses the scheme and allied skills related to the process as its basis, and the United Kingdom Central Council has indicated quite plainly that it expects all its nurses to use the technique.

As a result of this trend, I have not produced another 'psychiatry for nurses' book of which there are several good ones already on sale in this country. Instead, the book deals with the nursing process and explores its use and implications within the psychiatric discipline.

The content is a reflection of my own experiences and involvement and is largely based upon my teaching practice. It originated as a compilation of my teaching notes and was developed by working closely with the nursing staff on the psychiatric wards of the Norwich Health Authority, to whom I am eternally grateful. As a possible consequence of this, the reader may find it necessary to adapt what he reads to his own working situation. It must be remembered that this is only an approach to the subject. As more people implement the process, so the number of approaches will increase, but the process itself will always remain unchanged. This can only be good for psychiatry, which is largely misunderstood not only by the remainder of the nursing profession but by the lay population as a whole.

To some extent, we are fortunate in this country that we are only now beginning to tackle the process, because we have the opportunity to learn from the experience of others. Many of the ideas contained in this book would not have been possible had it been written twenty five years ago, when North America was beginning to outline the principles of the philosophy.

It is hoped that any differences of opinion that may manifest themselves during the reading of this book, between my own approach and those of the reader, will not inhibit the sense of excitement that the process brings. It is because the process enhances the amazing number of personal alternatives open to psychiatric nurses that the reader must develop his/her own individual style. In this way, it may become as successful and satisfying for him/her as it has for me, my colleagues and their patients.

Norwich, 1985   M.F.W.

Contents

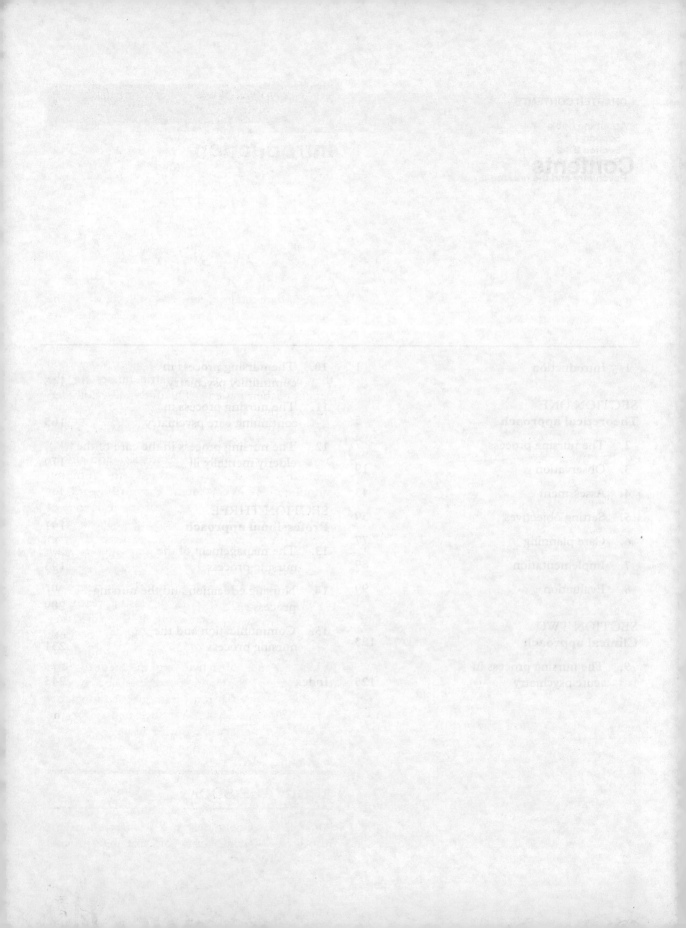

1

Introduction

The fundamental aspects and philosophy of the nursing process are the same whether they are used to deliver health care to premature babies, accident victims, cancer patients, cardiac cases, diabetics or the dying. The same is true when they are adopted by psychiatric nurses for the benefit of their patients. The difference, however, comes in their application in psychiatry.

Psychiatric nurses are responsible for a vast amount of independent nursing actions. They have at their disposal strategies and interventions which enable them to function autonomously. Very often, they will work for long periods of time away from the influence of other disciplines, thus having considerable impact on the progress of the patients. It is in this area of independence that the nursing process has its greatest part to play. Nurses must be given knowledge of, and experience in, using the skills of observing, assessing, planning, implementing and evaluating if the care they offer is to be truly effective. It has to be both scientific and artistic as well as holistically oriented and objective, complementing the treatment programmes prescribed by professional colleagues. It must be organised in such a way as to be realistic and therapeutic for the patient and manageable for the nurse.

ABOUT THE BOOK

This book has been designed to offer an insight into this special form of nursing process application for all grades of psychiatric nurses. The reader is provided with comprehensive and detailed information about the use of the process within a psychiatric framework. There are three sections within this book.

SECTION ONE

This section deals with the theoretical aspects of the process, taking each element in turn. It discusses various approaches and techniques that the nurse can use to accomplish a degree of competency, and applies them to an individual case study. This runs continuously through Chapters 3 to 8, eventually presenting a completed nursing process.

SECTION TWO

This section deals with the application of the nursing process in different areas of psychiatry: acute admission, community care, continuing care and the elderly mentally ill. Each is both a case study and a story, and views the responsibilities of constructing planned nursing intervention through the eyes of different members of the nursing team.

SECTION THREE

The final section deals with further applications of the process and considers educational and managerial approaches, communication activities, and the problems associated with change. The implications for the patient and the nurse form a major part of the section. Each chapter has a complete reference list and suggested reading list appropriate to the topics contained within the chapter. The reader must appreciate that a book of this nature can contain only a small fragment of the possible approaches that the nursing process offers the professional nurse, so further reading is essential.

PSYCHIATRY AND THE NURSING PROCESS

Although the nursing process is a philosophy of nursing appropriate to all the various disciplines and specialties, its suitability for psychiatry is unquestionably very great. No longer do thousands of lifeless individuals live empty lives, hounded by the sounds of bunches of keys and the slamming of locked doors. The bars on the windows have gone and so, too, the strait-jackets. The long-stay or continuing care population of the majority of psychiatric hospitals is an ever decreasing one and the needs of the staff are far more in line with current trends in human rights and community acceptance. Nurses are expected to keep pace with new ideas, both professional and social, which influence their role. Psychiatric nurses are now better educated than ever before; the academic qualifications required for training have increased, and the professional examinations are becoming more complex. The ability of nurses to assimilate more technical and complicated information about their patients and their behaviour has made them less tolerant of accepted practices. They are taught to question what is going on around them. Research into nursing practices has highlighted great gaps in existing approaches but very often has been unable to offer alternatives.

When a difficult situation develops on a busy ward, it is no longer simply a question of dealing with it by injecting those responsible with large doses of psychotropic medication. The situation has to be analysed and dealt with in a way that provides positive experiences for both the patients and the nurses. Both the profession and society expect and demand this, and anything less is regarded as undesirable.

Psychiatric nursing has, of course, many different facets and techniques. However, these facets usually centre around the concept of the nurse helping the patient to overcome some particular difficulty in his life. In other words, it is a question of problem-tackling. A person approaches his problems initially through a process of trial and error. Eventually, he learns to use a particular method to solve a particular problem. Each individual adopts his own methods and people recognise this. Consequently, he becomes categorised as being a particular type of person because he always behaves in certain ways when confronted with certain problems. This categorisation becomes what we call his personality. In more specific terms, the way the individual deals with the daily happenings of his life become stylised into the routine behaviour patterns. These patterns are usually directed towards reducing the anxiety he feels because of his problem. If he is successful in reducing, he will use that approach again in the future. The more stylised his behaviour becomes, the easier it is for others to categorise him. Thus, a person who always cries when distressed is regarded as being a 'depressive' by the lay population. Likewise, a person who is always immaculately dressed, with not a hair out of place, is regarded as being 'obsessional'. The personality of a person, then, is the way he behaves, or is perceived to behave. This behaviour becomes most apparent when he is under stress. If he has adopted an approach to solving his problems which only reduces, without dispelling, his feelings of anxiety, e.g. failing to attend an examination or avoiding a person who is angry with him, then in most situations the actual problem itself remains unresolved despite the reduction in anxiety. Continual use of this approach will deny him the satisfaction of real problem-solving, and the number of situations he can handle becomes more and more restricted. Ultimately, he may come into contact with psychiatric services, having stylised his behaviour so much that his anxiety-reducing strategies simply will not allow him the time to do anything else.

This is, perhaps, a rather simplistic view of psychiatric conditions but it is none the less an effective one. If the patient can be taught how to tackle the actual problem rather than dealing merely with the anxiety it provokes, he has a much better chance of being able to cope with similar problems in the future. By doing so, he will be better able to meet his daily needs, thus in turn reducing the feelings of frustration and stress that they create when left unsatisfied. In every sphere of psychiatric nursing, this theme of patient teaching is a constant one. With the aid of the nursing process, it is also a realistic one.

The nursing process helps the nurse to isolate those behavioural approaches used by a patient to protect himself from anxiety. It also enables her to examine the effect of the behaviour upon the individual's ability to function as an independent person. Finally, it helps the nurse to produce nursing intervention which will create a change in that behavioural pattern and enable the individual to develop his individual role once again. Of course, in some situations, it may be a question of slowing down a gradual deterioration in the individual's ability rather than helping to regain lost skills, as in the case of chronic brain failure. The basic principle, however, remains the same. The nursing process is designed to help the personality of the patient in a dynamic and systematic way such that it produces an increase in his problem-tackling ability.

The majority of care received by psychiatric patients comes from the nurse, and so it is particularly suitable that the nursing process should place so much emphasis upon the personalities of the parties who use it. If psychiatric nurses are to accept the challenge of new ideas, and offer their patients more effective intervention, they must adopt the philosophy of the process and use it at every possible opportunity.

The approach adopted in this book is consistent with the view that patients will never benefit fully from nursing intervention unless they are actively involved in it. If patients have no understanding of the method by which they managed to deal with a particular life problem, then the next time it arises, they are unlikely to deal with it successfully. Indeed, they may become more frustrated because they are aware that they have the capabilities to solve the problem and yet are apparently unable to do so. The nurse must realise that there is no set way to approach the nursing process, only the philosophy remains constant. The system by which it is adopted must be flexible and adaptable. The approach as outlined here, can be manipulated so that it can be used in any psychiatric situation. Having read the book, there is no reason why the nurse cannot then develop her own style as the process can often be a very personal thing. Most importantly, the process must be practised if it is to become effective.

SECTION 1
Theoretical approach

2

The nursing process

INTRODUCTION

Throughout history there have always been nurses, or at least someone who nursed. Some were paid for their skills; others merely did it out of the goodness of their hearts or because of family and group responsibilities. Their basic understanding of what they were doing was often quite limited and in some cases totally non-existent. Consequently, what they did for their patients was not always helpful and in many respects detrimental. The fact that many of those patients recovered was often due to their resilience rather than a tribute to those who cared for them. Gradually, as technology increased man's understanding of himself, nursing became a skilled activity with a more scientific approach. The nature of nursing, however, decreed that those innate, artistic qualities of human caring used in early times should still be incorporated into the general pattern. Nursing developed as an interplay between the two separate components of art and science. Unfortunately, the balance between the two became more and more difficult to regulate as technology grew. Eventually, it became necessary to train nurses in scientific areas and through that training nursing systems developed. These systems were designed to deliver high technology nursing to the patient whilst still maintaining the personal approach. In recent years, such systems as 'total patient care', 'the multi-disciplinary approach' and 'team nursing' have appeared and have then been superseded by others. The majority have been North American practices which have been adjusted to suit the United Kingdom health system. Unfortunately, because of the differences that exist between the basic health systems, these approaches, even when adapted, have been unsuitable or unmanageable. Because of this situation a general feeling of suspicion surrounds new nursing approaches which originate from America.

THE ORIGINS OF THE NURSING PROCESS

The nursing process also originated in America but unlike other systems it has stood the test of time and undergone continuous development since its conception. This is probably due to the fact that unlike other systems it does not restrict the nurse to rigid routines or procedures but provides her with a nursing philosophy based upon the principles of human needs. Strangely enough, its initial history remains something of a mystery. Orlando is credited with having first used the term, 'nursing process', whilst writing her book *The dynamic nurse patient relationship,* though she denies it. The actual need for the process grew out of the necessity of providing American medical insurance companies with a method of financially auditing the nursing care given to their clients. They needed to know how to price the care that was given and how often it would be given. Not until sometime later was it realised by a more enlightened nursing profession that this system also contained benefits of a nursing nature for those clients whilst they were still patients.

The nursing process evolved during the late 1950s and early '60s when much was changing within the American Health Care System and in the nursing profession as a whole. The emphasis in nursing shifted from simply giving care presented by other disciplines, to prescribing and managing care themselves and so the nursing process was born. Since those early days, the process has been adapted, enlarged and developed. It has become the basis of nursing itself and all new ideas or systems about nursing have incorporated its approach into their structure.

WHAT IS THE NURSING PROCESS?

Hargreaves (1979) described the nursing process as a combination of thought processes and nursing actions. A process, as Leonard and Redland (1981) point out, is any series of actions directed towards an objective. The nursing process, therefore, is a series of nursing actions directed towards the objective of patient health. The thought processes involved constitute a method of problem solving with certain definite steps. Each step must be successfully completed before the next in the sequence is attempted. It is the combination of the understanding required to complete each step and the actions they require for completion that make up the nursing process. The steps involved are very simple: observation, assessment, planning, implementation and evaluation. They are the same steps the individual uses to solve any problem, but usually he does so on an unconscious level. This means he is inclined to make mistakes. When he uses the same steps on a conscious level, thus taking into account all the various considerations available to him, analysing them, synthesising them and assessing them all in turn, he is less likely to make mistakes. The nursing process is therefore systematic because it follows a set pattern, and dynamic because it uses innate abilities on a conscious level. It is also a code of practice because it outlines a specific approach to problem tackling within a nursing sphere (De la-Cuesta 1983).

Which problem does it set out to tackle?

In psychiatry, the nursing process attempts to tackle the problems created by the expression of psychiatric illness. It does not try to solve the problem of, say, an hallucination, but rather attempts to solve the problem that hallucination creates for the individual who experiences it. It does not try to solve the problem of depression, but the problem or problems that depression creates for the individual who is depressed. In other words, when a person experiences a symptom of a psychiatric condition, it affects his ability to function as an independent person. He relies on someone else to help him deal with that situation. The nurse is that person. She must decide what problems that symptom is creating, then systematically decide on the best method to deal with them so that the patient can once again handle the situation for himself. If a person continually falls to the floor whenever he requires attention, the nurse must look at his communication patterns and establish a strategy for improving them. If a patient cannot dress himself, the nurse must find out why and then try to find a way to teach him to do so. If the patient is incontinent, the nurse must isolate the causes and devise a programme for achieving continence. The problems involved, then, are life problems. The nursing process looks at life problems and then designs ways of dealing with or adapting to them. It gives the nurse an insight into sometimes unexplainable patient behaviour through observation and assessment, then enables her to deal with the behaviour appropriately by planning and implementation. Finally, it evaluates what has been done to see whether or not the process has been effective.

A teaching element is also involved. It is not sufficient for the nurse simply to recognise a problem and deal with it herself. She has to find a way of devising care that will eventually teach the patient how to tackle that life problem for himself. If she fails to do this, then when the problem arises again, the patient will have no experience himself of the problem-tackling strategy and will, therefore, experience the same difficulties as before. It will then be necessary for the nurse to carry out the same nursing care once again and the patient will be no better off. The only way to achieve this teaching potential is to involve the patient in each of the problem-tackling stages and allow him to experience them for himself.

Bearing in mind all that has been said so far, a simple definition of the psychiatric nursing process is:

A systematic approach to tackling patients' life problems incorporating the steps of observation, assessment, planning, implementation and evaluation which enable the patient to solve, or adapt to, that problem himself (Ward 1988).

The words 'adapt to' are extremely important because in many situations, especially in psychiatry, it is almost impossible actually to solve these life problems. The individual may, rather, have to find a way of coming to terms with a continuing problem, thus giving him a degree of independence. For example, if a man has the desire to sexually expose himself, he is demonstrating a need for sexual expression. The method he has chosen conflicts with society's accepted norm and, therefore, creates stress for him. His problem is one of establishing a normal pattern of sexual expression. However, he is hampered by his shyness and lack of confidence and it seems unlikely that he will ever overcome these. In this situation, the nurse must try to teach him how to come to terms with a problem he may always have in such a way that he becomes more socially acceptable.

HOW DOES THE NURSING PROCESS WORK?

Having considered what the nursing process is, the next stage is to examine the way that it works. This is best achieved by outlining each of the five elements:

1. *Observation* of the patient in his total environment.
2. *Assessment* of the patient's needs.
3. *Planning* patient care.
4. *Implementation* of the patient's nursing intervention.
5. *Evaluation* of the suitability and effectiveness of the care plan.

Though the process can be divided into separate sections, this is an artificial separation because the whole process functions as a continuous and interdependent structure. Each stage follows on from the last and once the process has reached the evaluation stage, it starts all over again. It is thus a cyclical process, only complete when a problem is absolutely solved (Ward 1986).

OBSERVATION

The activity of observation is central to the whole concept of planned nursing, especially in a psychiatric context. It begins as soon as the patient arrives on the ward and does not stop until the day he is discharged. Even then, observation may well continue if he comes under the supervision of a community psychiatric nurse. It represents a systematic gathering and recording of all the necessary information about a patient relevant to the production and monitoring of his nursing intervention and medical treatment. Observation encompasses all functional aspects of the patient's behaviour, be they physical, psychological or sociological, and is called 'biopsychosocial observation'. In a world where attitudes and loyalties are constantly changing, younger nurses must also realise that this includes religious and spiritual beliefs. Information sources will include all those personnel who have had recent contact with the patient, as well as other nursing and medical colleagues. The main information source, however, is the patient himself, and the nurse must ensure that at all times he remains the key figure in her actions. Her observations must be objective rather than subjective. She must report facts, not her interpretation of those facts. She must avoid making judgements about what she sees or hears and she must also be aware of her own influence upon the patient's behaviour.

The nurse must be wary of collecting too much information. It becomes almost impossible to make accurate assessments about data if there are conflicting statements. Gathering of information irrelevant to the patient's treatment must be resisted. For example, a 69-year-old man suffering from the initial stages of chronic brain failure is admitted to the ward. The nurse, in her observations, gathers all the information from him that she possibly can, including details of the schools he attended, his military career and his childhood pursuits. These topics are ideal for reminiscence therapy or reality orientation but are hardly likely to assist the nurse in establishing the man's ability to wash and dress himself, or get to the toilet. The nurse's observations should not duplicate those of other disciplines involved in the care programme. If both the medical and nursing staff identify and report the same elements of patient behaviour, this is a serious waste of time. Nurses made

responsible for collecting data about a patient must, therefore, be aware of what has already been observed and reported. Basically, the nurse is trying to establish the effects of a patient's psychiatric condition on his ability to satisfy his own personal needs. This will mean establishing not only the overt or observable behaviour, but also the covert or hidden causes for that behaviour. She must find out why a patient feels he behaves the way he does, not just how he behaves. Within the structure of the approach to the nursing process outlined in this book, this is done by using straightforward non-participant observation called the 'nurse's impression' and a 'nurse's interview'.

It is vital that the information gathered about patient behaviour is recorded. This is done on progress notes and nurses' interview sheets. However, the initial response by the patient to hospitalisation is of special consideration and should be recorded on a sheet designed for this purpose. An example of this kind of admission record can be seen in Figure 2.1. It also incorporates relevant on-going data about the patient's stay in hospital, including a discharge plan. This record sheet is kept at the top of the patient's notes and provides the nurse with a constant reminder of the initial presentation.

The information, once recorded, forms the baseline from which the necessary decisions about nursing intervention and patient care objectives are made. They must, therefore, be complete, but not over-inclusive.

ASSESSMENT

Having gathered the information about the patient's behaviour, the nurse then has to make sense of it. This assessment will decide the direction in which the care will proceed. Obviously, a patient's nursing care begins as soon as he comes into contact with the nursing staff, and that initial care and the responses to it will constitute some guidelines for continuous nursing interventions. During this stage of the process, the nurse has to make three decisions. Firstly, she must decide from her observations which of the patient's basic human needs he is not capable of satisfying for himself and which, therefore, constitute problems. These problems may be obvious or they may be complicated to evaluate but it is essential that full consideration is given to all the facts available (Bergman 1983). Crow (1980) reported that nurses have great difficulty in establishing patient's problems and, in particular, those of a psychological or sociological nature. Physical problems, even for the trained psychiatric nurse, are often far easier to identify, but just as the observation process encompasses a biopsychosocial approach so too must the assessment. An example of this would be a list of personal problems which included:

- cannot wash himself
- cannot dress himself
- does not mix with others
- lacks personal confidence
- is afraid of his environment.

Secondly, the nurse must decide which of these problems she can deal with immediately and which will have to wait until resources and facilities become available. This is termed 'establishing need priorities'.

The third decision the nurse has to make is how best to express the need so that it relates to the patient's behaviour. For example: if the need to communicate satisfactorily with others is not being met, this could be for a hundred different reasons, from the patient having a poor grasp of the language to the fact that he is seated in a secluded corner. Therefore, the description of his need must be linked to his behaviour, for example, he fails to communicate with others because he shouts at people when they approach him. This statement is called the 'nursing diagnosis'. It differs from the medical diagnosis in that it relates the effect of a person's psychological condition to his ability to function independently, as opposed to isolating the psychological problem he is suffering from.

The patient must be involved in these three decisions. He must be helped to conceptualise his own difficulties even if he does not know their cause. This may be difficult with severely disturbed or disoriented patients, but they must still be offered the dignity of being allowed to influence their own care. The patient's interpretations of his problems may be at variance with

that of the nurse, but it must be given serious consideration if care is to be thought appropriate by both parties. This process of defining and agreeing on the problems with the nurse may well constitute the first stage of a patient actually learning to tackle problems for himself; this is, in effect, the whole purpose of the nursing process (Harden & Hales et al 1986).

PLANNING

Once the nursing diagnosis has been established, and there may be several different ones, the next stage is to decide what to do about them. Planning care involves two separate elements:

- setting objectives for the patient to achieve
- outlining the care necessary to achieve these objectives.

Once again, the patient must be involved in what is going on. It serves no purpose for him if care is thrust upon him without his consent or without his understanding of its purpose. Taking responsibility for decisions about his own care will enhance the patient's problem-tackling techniques. He must identify what he considers possible for him to achieve and the nurse should be able to tell him how she might help him to accomplish it.

The objectives will be either:

- short-term
- long-term.

The long-term objective for a specific nursing diagnosis is the eventual behaviour that the patient hopes to achieve with the aid of the nursing intervention. The short-term objectives are the small steps in between which eventually lead to the long-term objective. All of the short-term objectives must be achieved if the long-term objective is to be achieved successfully. Initially, only the long-term objective and the first of the short-term objectives need be agreed. The shape of the future short-term objectives will be dictated by the patient's progress.

The care outlined to achieve the objectives will, by virtue of her position, be essentially the responsibility of the nurse. She must use

Admission Sheet

Name:_____

Address:_____

_____

D.o.B. _____ Religion: _____

Marital status: _____

G.P. _____

Hospital _____ Ward _____

Consultant: _____ Next of kin:_____

Social worker: _____ Address: _____

Living alone/dependants: ____ _____

_____ Telephone No: _____

Pension book:_____ Relationship:_____

Valuables:_____ Admission status:_____

Height	Weight	TPR	Ward routine urinalysis

Admission nursing notes:

Date: _____

First night report:

Date:	Routine investigation:		Results:

Date:	Referrals:	Date:	Treatments:

Discharge plans: _____

Date of discharge: _____

Discharge address: _____

_____

Hospital car/ambulance arranged:_____ Yes/No _____

Medication given: _____ (_____days supply) _____

General practitioner's letter: _____ Given/Posted _____

Social worker notified:_____ Yes/No _____

Community nurse notified:_____ Yes/No_____ Name _____

Additional information:
e.g. Leaving against
medical advice, discharged—_____
from leave etc...

_____

Fig. 2.1B Admission sheet (reverse side).

accepted and established methods of care and not experiment with new ideas and techniques. This is because she must be aware of the effects of her intervention. She cannot afford to satisfy her own curiosity about experimental ideas at the expense of the patient's mental health.

Once the proposed care has been agreed by the patient, it is documented on the nurse's action sheet, or 'care plan' as it is called, along with the appropriate nursing diagnosis. Each nursing diagnosis, then, has its own objectives and its own carefully designed specific nursing intervention.

IMPLEMENTATION

Since the patient is already in hospital or in contact with psychiatric nursing personnel, he will already be receiving some form of nursing intervention. Once the care plan has been completed for his on-going care, that intervention may well be revised or continue as part of the programme. However, the specific elements of care outlined on the nursing care plan will constitute the basis of the patient's individual care and must be closely adhered to. Any deviation from the nursing required, any alteration or adaptation, will confuse the patient and reduce the effectiveness of the programme. If the patient has agreed to a certain approach and does not get it, or if he gets a variation of it, he may well become frustrated or disheartened. It makes little sense to gather all the relevant information, assess it and plan to do something about it, and then do something completely different.

EVALUATION

The fifth stage is that of evaluation. When the short-term objectives are set, a date is decided upon for their achievement. This gives both the patient and the nurse a target to aim for. This date becomes the time at which the programme is reviewed or evaluated. The nurse, in company with either her colleagues or the patient, decides whether or not they have been successful in achieving the short-term objective. This is done by considering three factors:

1. Does the patient's behaviour correspond with that laid down in the objective?
2. Was the nursing care given suitable for helping the patient behave in the required fashion?
3. Has the patient's presentation changed in such a way as to make the nursing diagnosis inappropriate?

Depending on the answers to these questions the care plan will need to be adjusted accordingly. If the objective is achieved, the patient and nurse decide on the next step. If, however, things have not gone according to plan, the patient must be helped to examine the causes and be involved in restructuring the approaches or reducing the objective. In both situations there should be a sense of movement along a recovery path that must be transmitted to the patient.

Once the evaluation procedure is complete, and new objectives and review dates are set, the whole cycle starts again. As problems are solved, needs met successfully and patient behaviour changing, so the pattern of care will alter accordingly. The eventual objective is that the patient is able to satisfy his own personal needs and thus become independent of the nurse. If, through her nursing intervention, the patient becomes dependent on the nurse, the nursing process has been only partially successful. When dealing with the elderly mentally ill, it may be necessary to accept such a limited success as the only possible outcome, but in most cases independence is the aim.

Observation and reporting of the patient's behaviour must be carried out throughout the process. Documenting data in his progress notes about his response to his care will provide the nurse with the tools for evaluation. Without that information, she cannot be expected to plan accurately the next stage in the patient's recovery or progress.

WHAT DOES THE NURSING PROCESS OFFER THE PATIENT?

If nursing is effective, it follows that what the patient receives from the nursing process must have great significance for him. In this instance, the word 'effectiveness' relates to the nurse's ability to identify and deal with the specific personal requirement of each individual patient in a way that creates independence. Further, the dignity offered the patient by being involved in the decision-making components of his nursing intervention provides a far more therapeutic environment than exists with traditional approaches to nursing. The whole purpose of using the nursing process is to give the patients better care. It is, therefore, necessary to isolate the main consequences of planned nursing intervention on the patient's experience of the care situation. These may be broadly described as:

- individualised nursing
- continuity of nursing intervention
- control within the intervention programme
- opportunity to choose alternative approaches
- motivation for progress
- dignity and self respect.

In some instances, not all of these consequences will be present. The elderly mentally ill may have little conception of the care that is being provided during the final stages of their life, but at least the process enables them to die with dignity. Patients of a continuing care nature may benefit from an improvement in their motivation. Initially, the patient may opt out of part of his care. However, all the nursing care will contain individuality and maintain continuity.

Individualised nursing

Each patient responds to his symptoms in a slightly different way. Ten patients with auditory hallucinations may have many common presenting features, but each one will be identified by his own particular mode of behaviour. Many factors contribute to this: environment, life experience, social and cultural background and physical make-up. Because each of these elements is unique to each of the patients, it makes sense that the care they are offered by the nurse must cater for this individuality. Providing nursing care entitled, 'Care of the patient with auditory hallucinations' fails to take these factors into consideration. The patients will require care which has basic similarities but their unique qualities must also be taken into account. Some patients are content to live with their symptoms and would, indeed, be lonely without them; others are deeply disturbed and distressed by them to an almost horrific extent. The ability of these patients and of their relations and friends to come to terms with the symptoms must be considered. The nursing process, by identifying the effects of the patients' responses to their symptoms in relation to their ability to meet their personal needs, offers an individualised approach to the care they should receive.

Within the nursing process, the framework for individualising care exists. When that individuality is transmitted to the patient, he becomes aware that his care has been devised especially for him. Someone has taken the time and the trouble to consider his particular problems and to design care that will help him. In effect, he becomes aware of his individuality more from a feeling of being cared about than being cared for.

Continuity of nursing intervention

Once care has been planned and negotiated with the patient, the next step is to implement it. The patient is fully aware of what is to happen and his expectations are consistent with that particular patient/nurse contract. If the continuity is interrupted in any way, this may produce doubt and uncertainty in his mind.

Continuity is all about the uninterrupted flow of planned nursing care. It means that if a patient has agreed, or in some cases been informed, that a plan of action will be followed, it will be so. Because it is written down, it does not matter whether or not the nurse with whom the patient made this contract is on duty. Nurses who are allocated the care plans of patients follow the same pattern of care delivery as those who conceived them. Should a nurse be drafted in from another area, she too will follow the same pattern. The patient receives the care designed to help him to reach his objectives until these objectives have indeed been reached.

The nursing process encourages nurses to carry out an uninterrupted sequence of pre-planned nursing actions. The patient expects them, and gets them. This continuity creates an environment where progress is potentially more achievable.

Control within the intervention programme

The nursing process sets out to involve the patient from the start. Consequently, progress is seen as a result not just of the nurse's action but also of the patient's own determination and effort. It gives the experience of problem-tackling that he needs and prepares him for future difficulties. Having an element of control is important because it gives a person self-identity and personal esteem. It allows for an element of reward to enter into the therapeutic situation. The patient feels a sense of responsibility and is motivated to take part in his nursing programme. A patient who experiences control, no matter how small, in his nursing intervention is a patient with a sense of purpose. Of course, patients who do not wish to be involved must also be allowed to make this decision, but should still be encouraged to take part as much as possible (Waterworth & Luker 1990).

Opportunity to choose alternative approaches

Self-expression comes in many forms but always centres around an element of choice. Just as it would be wrong to expect people to accept only a limited selection of personal goods in the shops, so too it is wrong to limit the nursing intervention available to them in a psychiatric hospital. It is also wrong to assume that all patients like the same type of intervention delivered in the same way. Finally, it is wrong to assume that the patient will accept care being delivered in the way that the nurse wants to offer it. Whenever possible, the nurse must seek alternative approaches to tackling problems and discuss them with the patient. Having done so, the patient should be given the opportunity to select the one he thinks is most suitable for him. In some situations, it may even be possible for him to construct a programme of his own under the guidance of the nurse. Allowing the patient this type of self-expression enables him to retain his personal identity.

Motivation for progress

The word 'motivation' has already been used to describe the effects of involvement and choice. Motivation is the desire to achieve a goal or satisfy a need. Without motivation, the individual lacks the necessary inducement to sustain his own life, and he dies. He dies because he does not meet his needs. In psychiatric hospitals, some patients lose their motivation through the institutionalisation process, some through the effects of outside pressure and some through personal failure. If the philosophy of the nursing process is adhered to by practising nurses and the patient is truly involved in planning, designing and choosing his own intervention programme, that motivation can be rekindled. It is the motivation to overcome his problems and meet his needs that will get the patient back to his rightful place in society.

Dignity and self-respect

Perhaps the most important element for every person, including both patient and nurse, is that of dignity. The whole concept of dignity can be seen in terms of pride or self-respect. It is derived from the way a person views himself and his own actions, and is expressed through his emotions. To be without dignity is to be without self-respect, and the psychological trauma that creates reduces a person's self-esteem and leaves him open to personal abuse. Sometimes a person's dignity is gauged by others because their actions signify respect or disrespect. Any action by one individual towards another which falls short of being respectful or proper is without dignity and, therefore, demeans the individuals involved.

The nurse, because of her unique position, can easily reduce a patient's dignity simply by leaving him unscreened whilst he uses a commode, by making cynical remarks about him behind his back or by ignoring him completely. These things cannot be altered by the nursing process because they are a matter of the nurse's own integrity. However, the simplest way of producing an undignified patient is for the nurse to treat the patient as a child. This can be rectified by the nursing processes. Children are very rarely given the opportunity to make real decisions about themselves. As they grow older and more knowledgeable so this responsibility is encouraged until they are grown up and take full responsibility for their own decisions and for the consequences of those decisions. If the patient is involved and active in his own care his dignity will remain intact and feelings of inferiority will not obstruct his progress.

SUMMARY

The nursing process has evolved because of a need to make nursing more effective, both for nurses and patients. Florence Nightingale (1859) was probably the first person to outline this concept and today it has become the accepted philosophy for enlightened nurses throughout the world (Henderson 1987). It is a systematic approach to problem-tackling which involves both patient and nurse in a series of actions designed to produce individualised nursing interventions. It is not a system of nursing but a philosophy which is dynamic and adaptable. It is particularly suited to psychiatric nursing because it requires the nurse to examine her patients on a biopsychosocial level. By its usage, each patient is treated as an individual with his own special requirements and needs, and he is given the opportunity to become involved in the production and direction of his own intervention programme.

REFERENCES

Bergman R 1983 Understanding the patient in all his human needs. Journal of Advanced Nursing 8: 185–190
Crow J 1980 The effects of preparations on problem solving. Royal College of Nursing, London
De la-Cuesta 1983 The nursing process: from development to implementation. Journal of Advanced Nursing 8: 365–371
Hargreaves I 1979 Theoretical considerations. In: Kratz C K (ed) The nursing process. Baillière Tindall, London, Ch.1
Harden J, Hales R E et al 1986 In-patient participation in treatment planning: A preliminary report. General Hospital Psychiatry 8(4): 287–290

Henderson V 1987 The nursing process in perspective–Guest editorial. Journal of Advanced Nursing 12: 657–658
Leonard B J, Redland A R 1981 Process in clinical nursing. Prentice Hall, New Jersey
Nightingale F 1859 Notes on nursing. Harrison and Sons, London. 1946 J B Lippincott Co, Philiadelphia
Ward M F 1986 Learning to care on the psychiatric ward. Hodder and Stoughton, Sevenoaks
Ward M F 1988 The nursing process. In: Krebs M J S, Larsen K H (eds) Applied psychiatric-mental health nursing standards in clinical practice. John Wiley, New York, Ch.1
Waterworth S, Luker K A 1990 Reluctant collaborators: do patients want to be involved in decisions concerning care? Journal of Advanced Nursing 15(8): 971–976

SUGGESTED READING

Rhodes B 1985 Occupational ideology and clinical decision making in British nursing. International Journal of Nursing Studies 22(3): 69–75
Richards D A, Lambert P 1987 The nursing process: the effects on patient satisfaction with nursing care. Journal of Advanced Nursing 12(5): 559–562

Robinson D 1990 Two decades of the process. Senior Nurse 10(2): 4–6
Shields P J, Morrison P 1988 Consumer satisfaction on a psychiatric ward. Journal of Advanced Nursing 13: 396–400
Walton I 1986 The nursing process in perspective. Department of Social Policy and Social Work. University of York, York

3

Observation

INTRODUCTION

The initial phase of the nursing process is that of observation – the gathering of relevant information about the patient's ability to function as an independent person which enables the nurse to formulate nursing intervention consistent with the patient's real needs. This will help him to become independent of the nurse rather than dependent upon her.

It is absolutely vital that positive as well as negative elements in the presentation are observed and reported, which means that a systematic approach is required. Only by observing accurately can the nurse hope to individualise the care provided. Effective psychiatric nursing relies heavily on the ability of the nurse to gain information about her patients because perhaps as much as 90% of all health care delivered will be of a nursing nature. Case histories taken by doctors, social workers, psychologists and occupational therapists will reflect their own commitment to the patient in relation to what they are capable of offering. What nurses are interested in is finding out how those symptoms affect the individual in his daily life. The information collected by nurses should thus complement, rather than duplicate, that gathered by other disciplines connected with the patient. In this way, a patient profile will develop related to what the psychiatric nurse can offer.

OBSERVATION

The role of the psychiatric nurse can be defined as:

1. Teaching patients how to tackle those problems in their own environment which inhibit their ability to function independently of others

   or, if this is impossible or unrealistic,

2. Helping those patients to develop personal strategies which will enable them to come to terms with their own level of function.

For example, we may need to know whether Peter's active delusional system prevents him from interacting with those around him, thus denying him his need to socialise. Does it inhibit his judgement of his surroundings, creating for him a hostile environment and thus denying him his needs for personal safety and security? Does it stop him from eating regular meals and drinking adequate amounts of fluids, thus denying him his very basic needs of food and water? The questions are as endless as the lists of individual needs, but it is only through observing the effect of the symptoms (i.e. the patient's behaviour) that the nurse will be able to identify those needs which are not being met.

Abilities as well as disabilities must be noted. A list showing needs that are not being satisfied implies that total inability exists, but when weighed against a list of needs that are being satisfied it offers useful information about the patient's present ability, potential ability and levels of personal gratification. It also indicates how much the individual may be able to help himself and pinpoints those areas that will require the specialist help of the nurse.

For example, at 15 years of age Susan may be failing to come to terms with her changing body image, her role in society, her relationship with her parents, her sexuality and that of others. She may have stopped eating and be reduced to a body weight of only 32 kg, thus denying herself the satisfaction of any number of biopsychosocial needs; however, she can wash and dress herself, and

socialise with her peers, appreciate pop music and the attention offered her by her treatment programme. She is not without personal satisfaction and, therefore, not totally dependent.

It will be noticed that at no time has the word 'assessment' been mentioned. This is intentional, for although observation and assessment are closely linked, they are still separate. Most authorities, when discussing the nursing process, link the two together, but for the psychiatric nurse this is a potentially dangerous method of establishing care essentials. If the nurse were told that over a period of time it had been noted that George would not eat meat at any time and that if he did so inadvertently he would vomit fiercely, that he would always choose dairy products at meal times, that he would not vomit after eating any other form of food, that there was no evidence of gastric dysfunction and that he stated he had been a life-long vegetarian, she would be quite right to conclude that this was the case. If the same nurse were told that Mabel could not get up out of bed and she stated that she was too old to do so and her bones ached, the nurse would be wrong to assume that Mabel was too feeble to do anything for herself and therefore needed all activities of daily living to be done for her, in addition to receiving passive physiotherapy. Why? Because Mabel might be quite capable of doing these things physically, but has lost the motivation to do so. The nurse made an assumption based on incorrect data, rather than drawing a conclusion from all available sources.

An assumption is the worst form of decision to arrive at, and if nurses formulate unprofessional assumptions about their patients long before they have gathered all the relevant information together they may be responsible for the implementation of totally inadequate and inappropriate nursing intervention. In other words, the nurse must look hard before acting.

One example of this is the newly admitted patient who sits with his wife in the day area. When she prepares to leave he becomes tearful and distressed. His nurse helps the wife to leave and then consoles the patient by saying, 'Don't worry, she will be back to see you'. This approach is used to console the man for the remainder of the shift and is only challenged when the night nurse notices that it has little effect. When she questions the patient she discovers that he was crying *because* his wife was returning and he could not bear for her to see him in such a terrible state. This sad man had been tormented throughout the day because of a thoughtless assumption.

Perhaps more seriously, but of a similar nature there is the unfortunate anecdote of the patient who told the psychiatrist he was being followed everywhere. The psychiatrist instantly placed the man on major tranquillisers and advised everyone on his team that the patient was suffering from paranoid delusions. It transpired several weeks later that the man's wife, being outrageously jealous and suspecting infidelity, had indeed hired a private detective to trail her husband. A blunder of such magnitude would never have arisen had the correct observation policy been adopted. Observation is a passive pursuit, passive in so far as no active conclusions are made about the information gathered until sufficient has been collected to allow accurate statements to be made. It may involve actively controlling the environment in which the patient finds himself, but it remains passive from a decision-making point of view.

OBSERVATION CRITERIA IN PSYCHIATRY

Just what is it that psychiatric nurses need to observe? Here we meet several conflicting arguments. Some authors say that all factors relating to the patient in his total environment should be noted (Marriner 1979, Kron 1981, Jukes 1987) while others say that it is far better to observe functions rather than symptoms (Smith 1980, Miller 1984, Peterson 1987). It is necessary to do both but to emphasise the functional aspect by illustrating it with the symptomatic background. Nurses need to be able to identify the specific requirements of their patients and can only do this by measuring their levels of personal effectiveness. It is of little value to have a record of abilities and disabilities. What acade-

mic studies cannot hope to tell the nurse is how each one of these various elements is going to affect the patient's ability to control his own life. The 'symptom' may not be a clinical one either, but part of a sociological sequela that inhibits true adaptability. It may be a physical dysfunction that can only be rectified using medical strategies. It may be a psychological phenomena, real only to the individual who experiences it. In all these cases, no matter what the origin of the symptom or the symptom itself, there is always a requirement for a nursing intervention.

During the last 25 years much has been published on observational criteria. The vast majority of this has dealt with the patient receiving care in the general hospital setting. Some of this is appropriate to the psychiatric discipline. The work of Roper et al (1981) includes a modified version of Hendersons Activities of Daily Living (1960). Roper's list includes:

- maintaining a safe environment
- communicating
- breathing
- eating and drinking
- eliminating
- personal cleansing and dressing
- controlling body temperature
- mobilising
- working and playing
- expressing sexuality
- sleeping
- dying.

Abdullah's (1960) list of 21 nursing problems, and Geitgey's (1969) SELF PACING are other methods that have been used. Unfortunately, the problem with using these methods in the psychiatric discipline is that they do not offer the scope needed to establish both overt and covert patient needs as indicated by Abdullah in her earlier research (1957). Covert needs are those patient problems which are concealed but which may have displaying symptoms. The majority of nursing observation criteria deal with overt patient problems, i.e. those aspects of patient problems with obvious, or seemingly obvious, causes.

For example; an overt problem for George may well be the fact that he cannot eat meat;

therefore, the nurse must ensure that he has sufficient alternatives and receives a balanced diet. The covert problem for George might be the fear or apprehension that he will be made to eat meat whilst in hospital because there is no alternative. The function of the nurse here is to make him aware of the alternatives and help him select those he would most enjoy, whilst ensuring that he is totally aware that he does not have to eat anything he does not want to, that he will receive a balanced diet and that all the staff are aware of the situation. In other words, a total approach to both the overt and covert aspects of the same problem is necessary. This covert/overt element must be included in any observational pattern that is used to constitute observational criteria.

There is no need to produce a medical biography of the patient nor one of scant reference, but rather what Williams called the 'patient profile' (Williams 1960).

This begins with a brief but relevant summary of the patient's life events and his response to them for the period up to his admission, transfer or hospitalisation. The nurse needs to know how the patient has adapted to his hospitalisation and what his expectations of this hospitalisation are. She needs to know his feelings as to why he is receiving care and what he hopes to achieve before discharge, and after. These, and many other questions will form the basis of the patient profile which eventually will help the nurse to help the patient help himself. None of the staff from other disciplines who will be involved with the patient will have such a total approach to him, and this is why the initial observations and records are so important for his personal progress.

NURSING METHODOLOGY

The psychiatric observation process can be broken into two main parts:

1. The nurse's impression of the patient in his clinical environment and that information gained from other sources which will be used as a functional comparison.
2. The nurse's interview.

THE NURSING IMPRESSION

It must be emphasised that the observation process is not an exercise in spying on the patient but a mutual activity of involvement. The patient must be made to feel that he is participating in his own care, that he is not being enveloped in the cloak of apparent mystique which seems to surround psychiatry, nor that attempts are being made to trick him in some way. Trust is one of the basic elements of real communication and a pattern of mutual trust must be initiated here in the observation section.

INFORMATION SOURCE

The information source is that point at which related behavioural activity data is gained. It will vary from ward to ward and clinical area to clinical area. The major source is the patient himself. He alone has the key to his own functional ability. Close observation is necessary not only of the patient himself, but also of the parts of his environment with which he is in contact. The following are the observational elements required most.

Observational elements

1. How does he behave whilst on the ward?

This is a general impression of the major behavioural presentation and a statement about the physical manifestations of his emotional difficulties and conflicts.

2. How does he respond to his fellow patients?

No person lives in a vacuum. He may withdraw from them, appear to be suspicious of them or be frightened of them. He may select certain people to sit with and talk to, or he may become angry or agitated in the company of others. Who are his friends and do they fit into a specific type of group, i.e. young, old, disturbed, capable, efficient, prepared to help him, quiet or gregarious?

3. How does he respond to the staff?

Are there any particular staff members to whom he seems able to relate? Is he dependent, or independent? Does he ignore them or seek them out? Does he relate better to his fellow patients? Does his mood change in their presence?

4. How does he socialise?

This is a general statement but it should be qualified by examples of how he behaves in set circumstances. Is he withdrawn or does he mix well?

5. What questions does he ask of the staff/patients?

This will give a good indication as to what is uppermost in his mind and not what the nursing staff feel he should be thinking.

6. Does he leave the ward?

Where does he go and with whom? How does he seem when he leaves and on his return? Is there anything which occurs on the ward which precedes his departure from it?

7. Is he able to orient himself to his surroundings?

Is he disoriented; if so, how? Does he find his environment a threat? Does he know where to find the toilet, the TV or radio, the lounge, his bed, the kitchen, the nursing station and the dining area?

8. Does he seem interested in himself?

How does he dress? Is he smart or untidy? Does he attend to his personal hygiene? Does he shave or does she wear make-up?

9. Does he appear interested in his care?

Is he preoccupied with his own problems or has he managed to avoid them?

10. Is he dependent or independent?

How much do the nurses do for him? How much does he ask them to do? Does he get other patients to help him? Does he ask to be helped or does he use other methods of gaining attention which are less acceptable?

11. What is he able to do for himself?

How does he occupy himself? Is he occupied or preoccupied? Does he seem to be more at peace when actively involved in the ward, or in ward activities? Is he more at peace when quiet or unoccupied? Does he make his own bed, get his own drinks and serve himself at mealtimes?

12. Does he have any physical pain?

Does he complain of pain, biologically identified or otherwise? Does he request pain-killers?

13. Does he eat well?

Does he eat all his meals; if so what does he eat? Does he appear to enjoy his food, or is he simply going through the motions? Does he have any particular favourites in his diet?

14. Does he eliminate regularly?

A bowel chart is not always necessary, just a simple check on his visits to the toilet unless otherwise indicated. Is fluid balance appropriate? Does he experience difficulty in voiding? Is he constipated? Has he any pain or discomfort? Does he ask for aperients?

15. Does he sleep well?

The night staff will make comments about his sleep pattern on his first night of admission and use this as a baseline for further information. Does he sleep during the day; if so, when?

16. Does he have any physical problems?

Has he any physical handicap that might inhibit him in his bid to be independent. Does he have a walking aid, a hearing aid, spectacles? If so, does he use them? Is he capable of independent mobility?

17. Do his clinical symptoms affect his ability to be independent?

Clinical symptoms cannot be ignored but how do they affect him? Can he cope with their effect? Do his cognitive processes function correctly, allowing him to concentrate, converse, relax or understand? The list is as long as the symptoms he may be experiencing. In many respects, it will be his anxiety that inhibits his ability to solve his own problems, both environmental and personal.

18. Does he have visitors?

Yes or no? How do these visitors affect him? Is he pleased to see them and does he enjoy their company or does he become irritable and argumentative? How does he seem when they have departed? Does he discuss the visits?

19. When does he appear most satisfied?

Look for positive elements in his behaviour, not just negative ones.

20. Under what circumstances does his behaviour change?

No patient's mood remains constantly stable, even if he is deeply depressed. When is he relaxed, disturbed, aggressive, happy, anxious, apprehensive, cheerful, bright or distressed?

21. Does he appear to be a threat to himself or others?

Is he a danger to himself? Has he self-destruct intent? Is he able to identify the dangers in the environment, or is his judgement poor or suspect? Is he at risk when left alone? Does he threaten others; if so, why, when, and who?

22. How has he changed since admission?

This is an important area because it will indicate the effect of his change of environment. Is he more relaxed and at peace or is he more disturbed and less likely to be able to lead an independent life?

It must be remembered that the above is not exhaustive of the observations that might be made, but they should form the nucleus of any observational impression made by the nurse. They do not involve asking questions of the patient on a formal basis, but it will be necessary to verify the observations with him, especially if they are causing either distress or disturbance.

The methods of gaining this information are both varied and simple. They involve any number of the following activities and information sources:

1. Reading:
   - case notes of previous admissions
   - medical case notes on admission and subsequent entries
   - social histories
   - family doctor referrals
   - social service referrals
   - domiciliary reports
   - occupational therapy reports
   - nurse's progress notes
   - treatment progress sheets.

It must be remembered that any psychiatric admission, especially to the acute areas, may be a re-admission. Extensive comparison information about the patient should therefore be available. This can be verified against current behavioural patterns and possibly reduce observational times.

2. Being aware of the patient's location throughout the shift. This does not involve constant checking or spying. The nurse could ask the patient to keep her informed of his whereabouts if he intends to leave the ward; and whilst on the ward, unless his behaviour warrants special attention, he should be free of constant overt nursing supervision.

3. Talking to visitors and relatives about the patient's usual behaviour and his general

approach to solving his daily problems. This information can be compared with the current picture.

4. Discussing the patient's response to his admission with those personnel who were in any way involved with it, i.e:

- ambulance teams
- social workers
- police
- community psychiatric nurses
- hospital porters/ancillary staff.

5. Seeking the advice of colleagues and using their observational skills both in the nurse's absence and as a comparison for her own findings.

6. Spending as much time as possible with the patient in activities of both a clinical and a non-clinical nature. The nurse should avoid giving the impression that the only times she wishes to approach the patient is when she wants something from him. This will destroy his confidence in her and cloud the issue of her intent. She must show that she is interested in him as a person and not simply as a 'case'. This also involves joining patient groups with which he is associated, both formal and informal.

7. Observing the effect that the patient has on other staff members and patients alike. The nurse should ensure that she never asks questions concerning her patient of other patients. Not only will this have a harmful effect on her relationship with that patient should he ever receive knowledge of her enquiries, but it may also reduce her credibility amongst the remainder of the patient group.

8. Monitoring the following clinical progress data:

- nursing care records
- voiding tables/times
- bowel charts
- continence records
- turning charts
- skin condition/pressure area risk cards
- mood swing flow charts
- sleep pattern charts
- occupation records

- diet sheets
- anxiety flow charts
- orientation graphs
- conversation records
- mobility/activity records.

It is obvious that the information sources listed above represent only a cross-section of those available to the psychiatric nurse. On some wards many of them may be part of the resources present and in others there may be more that can be used. It must be stressed that it would be unrealistic to expect to gain information from all these sources. It would be both time consuming and, in many respects, provide totally useless data. The nursing impression is not intended to be a data bank of unlimited size, but an indication of the salient factors in the individual's presentation which indicate areas on a personal level for which adequate nursing intervention can achieve a degree of improvement or adaptation. The patient must be aware of the observations and be involved in the identification of behavioural patterns or significant causes for altered presentations. He must be asked about his feelings after observed events, and the insignificance for him.

The initial observation of a patient involves a very large commitment from the nurse assigned to carry out the work. If these first few days are interrupted by days or periods off the ward, then a substitute nurse must be found so that an element of consistency and continuity is achieved. It is never advisable to have more than two nurses made responsible for this initial activity as this may give rise to conflicting reports and consequent confusion. Appropriate information can be plotted in the initial nursing progress notes. The base line observational material from which the nursing diagnosis will be made should be placed on a separate sheet headed 'Nursing impression' and placed in the nursing progress notes as soon as possible to avoid any lapse in communication. Whenever possible, information should not be duplicated, i.e. the information that appears in the progress notes should not also appear as part of the nursing impression.

THE NURSE'S INTERVIEW

The type of interview used will be of a semi-structured nature. Open-ended questions are put to the patient so that he has an adequate opportunity to express himself within a working framework. In recent years, there has been an increase in patient questionnaires, tick lists and data sheets for the purpose of interviewing but these are not always suitable for the psychiatric discipline. Their formal structure does not allow any adaptability and all patients are asked the same questions. This is either time consuming or irrelevant to many patients. In psychiatry, the interview should offer the patient the kind of involvement in his own care that will allow him to feel that he has some control over what happens to him, and that the nurses with whom he comes into contact are working with him, and not for him or despite him. The taking of complex social, cultural and mental state histories has no place here either, as these are usually taken by other team members working with the patient. A patient will soon lose confidence in a care team which constantly asks the same questions without ever seeming to act upon his answers.

Observational criteria

The interview will include those questions not already answered by the nurse's impression. The following constitute the basis of those questions:

1. What does the patient expect from being in hospital?
2. How does he experience his own illness?
3. Why does he feel that he has been admitted?
4. What are his impressions of his hospitalisation?
5. What does he expect from the nursing staff?
6. What does he feel capable of doing for himself?
7. How do his psychiatric symptoms affect his ability to function as he would wish?
8. Has he any awareness of his condition, situation or behaviour?
9. How does he cope with his activities of daily living?

10. What influence do his relatives or visitors have upon him?
11. What is troubling him most at present?
12. What would he most like to be able to do at present?
13. What influence has the hospitalisation process had upon him?
14. What does he feel his potential for progress and rehabilitation is?
15. How does he see his future?

The formulating of a suitable set of questions will depend on several factors:

- the kind of ward
- the patient's level of ability and awareness
- the facilities that can be offered
- the expected duration of patient stay
- the baseline level of competence shown by the patient
- what has already been established in the nursing impression.

Each clinical area should decide on the type of questions it needs to have answered and give priority to those that it feels are of most significance. For example, in the case of the elderly psychiatric patient, the staff may give priority to the patient's ability to carry out activities of daily living, and in the continuing care area to how the symptoms affect the individual's performance and potential. The interview must therefore be flexible and adaptable. It is totally wrong to expect the same set of questions to be applicable to all patients, as stereotyped questions will produce stereotyped answers and stereotyped care. This practice is contrary to the principles of the nursing process.

Constructing the interview

Staff in the clinical area should have a list of the basic observational criteria and decide what they can deal with best. Certain items are indispensable, such as the patient's feelings about his ability and his hospitalisation, and even in situations where the staff feel that he may not be able to answer these questions, as with disoriented, disturbed and withdrawn individuals, he must be offered the chance to do so. From the basic list, the senior ward staff in consultation with their nursing teams should decide for each separate patient those interview questions that will most highlight the nature of the patient's personal problems and those which staff are suitably equipped to deal with. Questions themselves do not necessarily need to be constructed at this time but could be left to the interviewing nurse at the time of the interview.

As Figure 3.1 shows, a nursing interview sheet consists of the following:

- the patient's full name
- the patient's preference for what he likes to be called
- his clinical area or ward
- his hospital number
- the date or dates that the interview took place
- space for writing the interview record
- space for recording the nurse's general impression of the patient during the interview.

In the space for the interview record, the nurse should head each section with the observational criteria that she is hoping to gain information about, or the specific questions she asks the patient. All the items required should be noted to give those using the sheet as a reference a guide as to what it contains. The patient's responses to the questions should be entered underneath.

The completed form must always be signed by the nurse carrying out the interview: (1) to ensure reference to the individual concerned and (2) as validation of the information it contains. The area marked 'General impression of the patient during interview' at the end of the sheet gives the nurse the opportunity to record non-verbal responses to the interview.

Interview activity

Because the nurse has to think about and construct the questions herself, they should have more significance for both parties. There is nothing more abhorrent than a nurse sitting before a frightened or disturbed person asking a series of neverending questions from a list in front of her. Such an action can only convey the feeling that the nurse is more interested in the checklist than in the patient, especially if there is no room to record answers to questions she did not ask.

It is essential that only trained staff or senior learners carry out the nurse's interview. Nursing or care assistants, like the junior learner, have neither the training nor the background scientific knowledge to be able to cope with this nursing activity and should therefore not be asked to carry it out.

The questions themselves are obviously of great importance. They must not contain the easy answer in their own make-up (Peplau 1960, Elder 1978, Bunch 1985), nor must they be too restrictive or so specific as to inhibit the patient's self-expression. For example, having admitted a patient to the ward it is decided that three points in his presentation need to be clarified.

1. What does the patient expect from being in hospital and from the nursing staff?
2. How do his psychiatric symptoms affect his performance or ability to function?
3. What is his potential for progress and rehabilitation?

The interview covering these areas could contain the following care questions:

Questions

- Why have you come to this hospital?
- How do you feel the nurses here can help you?
- What would you like the nurses who help you to do?

There could be an interlude here whilst the modern role of the nurse is discussed, as patients often have misconceived ideas about this. Helping the individual achieve independence in areas of inability could also be mentioned, thus facilitating further discussion at a later date.

Questions

- Tell me about your day when you are at home.
- How do you think your day will change whilst you are in hospital?

Nurse's Interview

Full Name: _____

Clinical area: _____

Interview date(s): _____

Interview:

Item

response

Item

response

Item

response

Item

response

Item

response

Name preference: _____

Hospital number: _____

Nurse's signature: _____

Fig. 3.1A   Nurse's interview.

Side two

Item

response

Item

response

Item

response

Item

response

Item

response

General impression of patient during interview(s)

Fig. 3.1B Nurse's interview (cont'd).

● Tell me about the people you see during your day.

These questions should elicit a picture of the individual's own perception of his daily routine, his social contact and his activities.

Questions

● What would you like to be able to do for yourself if it were at all possible?
● Do you think the staff will be able to help you achieve these aims?
● Is there anything that you know of that has stopped you from achieving these things in the past?

A brief discussion here about the patient's involvement in his own care, his commitment to the treatment programme, the setting of objectives, and the acquisition of new personal strategies should contribute to his understanding of the situation. It might give him a clearer view of his role as a patient.

Questions

● Tell me about those things in your life which make you feel most happy.
● How do you feel about life at the moment?
● What do you hope to do when you leave hospital?

The dialogue should finish with the patient feeling that the interview has had both a beginning and an end. He should also feel that not only has he contributed to it but that he has gained something from it.

Where more areas need to be investigated, fewer core questions may have to be used to ensure that the interview does not become an unwieldy mass of words too complicated for accurate interpretation. Often, one question can provide the answers to many others so the nurse must avoid being over inclusive.

Patient responses

The patient responses can be recorded in one of two ways:

1. short phrases or sentences used by the patient
2. a summary of what was said.

The first of these is probably the most effective method because only the words used by the patient are recorded, thus avoiding the possibility of the nurse making subjective comments about her material.

Time span

The initial interview should be carried out in the first week of admission. It may be done over a period of several days if necessary, but should not be started before the patient has had time to orientate himself to the change in his environment. The interview differs from the nursing impression in that the nurse is not trying to gauge the patient's responses to his situation. A period of 48 hours should elapse before the interview is initiated. If the nurse who undertakes the interview is the same nurse who admitted the patient, this will increase the possibility of the patient/nurse relationship reaping early benefits for both parties.

In the case of patients being re-admitted, old notes should not be used as a baseline, as the patient profile should relate to the current situation. Obviously, detailed nursing and medical notes will provide first class background data but they may not always be applicable a second time around.

INFORMATION STORAGE

On a ward where there is a large patient population, much writing and paperwork will accumulate over a period of time. It is essential that the data collected from the observational period is stored in a system from which it can be easily retrieved. It is suggested that the interview sheet constitute the second part of the patient's profile (the first being the top sheet discussed in Chapter 2). It must be stressed that, where possible, the writing should be kept to an absolute minimum. Only relevant information should therefore be recorded. Repetition and subjective statements have no place here.

The practice of observing patients is one with which all nurses are familiar, especially in the psychiatric discipline. Being more objective about those observations can only improve the nurse's effectiveness. It is necessary, however, to see how the technique described can be applied to the pratical situation. We will, therefore, consider the application of the observation strategies within a case study. The study is taken from the acute admission area, and contains a brief resume of the patient, a nursing impression and the nurse's interview.

CASE STUDY: JULIE DAWSON

BACKGROUND

Julie Dawson is a 23-year-old secretary with a large building firm. She is a bright, intelligent young woman, well qualified and, according to her employers, very good at her job. Recently, there has been a marked deterioration in her work, with poor attendance, bad time keeping and a host of small errors which have created much work for her colleagues. She is described as a quiet girl with no close friends at work, though she is always cheerful and well accepted. Prior to this deterioration in her work, she was offered the possibility of a further training course which would have meant promotion for her. She turned this down. She has not attended work for three weeks.

Julie lives at home with her elderly parents and is an only child. Both are well and father still works as a clerical officer. Neither have a history of psychiatric problems. They describe their daughter as being somewhat shy and unassuming with very little social life. Her main interests appear to be reading and music, and she plays the guitar, though only to herself. She maintains contact with one or two of her old school friends but rarely goes out at night. To the best of her parents' knowledge, Julie has not had a steady boyfriend since leaving school, though she has been out with several boys over the intervening years.

During the last few months, Julie has become less communicative than before, spending much of her time in her own room doing very little. On several occasions mother thinks she has heard her daughter talking to someone in an angry voice, during the night, but there has never been anyone else in the house. She has been doing less and less around the house, and her usual neat appearance has become rather neglected. She refuses to cook for herself and will not carry out household chores, something she has always done eagerly in the past. She has taken to spending all her weekends in bed, and 2 weeks ago went to bed and has refused to rise ever since.

When spoken to she mumbles in response and much of what she actually says seems non-sensical. Eventually the local doctor was called, and having examined Julie requested a visit from the psychiatrist. He suggested Julie should be admitted to hospital for close observation and, though reluctant to leave her bed, she agreed.

It took nearly 48 hours for her actually to arrive at the hospital, mainly because she could see no reason for doing so. She finally concluded that this was a divine mission and in the company of her mother and a female social worker presented for admission.

ON ADMISSION

Julie did not speak at all on admission, except to bless the admitting nurse and the social worker. The ambulance crew who brought her said she had blessed them also whilst in transit. She was dressed in a nightdress and house coat and looked unkempt and dishevelled. Her nails were dirty, as were her feet and she refused to wear slippers. Her hair was greasy and knotted. She did not appear to take any interest in her surroundings and would answer no questions put to her. She did not appear to understand where she was, though this could not be confirmed because of her lack of communication. A cup of coffee offered her was blessed by her then thrown around the nursing station. She remained calm, withdrawn and uncommunicative throughout her admission.

FIRST WEEK

No fresh information appeared during this period. Julie refused most meals, unless she could have them in bed where she continued to spend most of her time. Several hours had to be spent coaching her to pay attention to the basics of her personal hygiene and she would sit up straight in bed all the time, refusing to sleep for as long as possible. She slept for only 7 hours during the first 5 days. Everyone who attended her was blessed by her, and she requested, and was given, a bible which she never read but always carried and made reference to. Fluid intake was poor and she had no bowel activity. She had no awareness of her surroundings and it was evident that auditory hallucinations were taking up much of her time. She could not hold a mutual conversation, never initiated discussion and found great difficulty concentrating for even small periods of time. Though having nurse contact practically all the time, she formed no relationship with any of her nurses, often not being able to remember them despite considerable familiarity.

THE NURSE'S INTERVIEW

Several points about Julie's presentation are very noticeable:

1. her attention to activities of daily living
2. her awareness of her surroundings and their implications for her
3. how she experiences her own condition
4. what she expects of those around her.

These areas will constitute the basis of her interview (Figs 3.2 and 3.3).

This young girl is obviously experiencing severe psychological disturbance which has dramatically affected her ability to lead a satisfying coexistence with her environment. Her dependence on the staff is almost total. During the nurse's impression and interview, psychological, sociological and biological difficulties have been identified in relation to her present condition and that of her previous history. Both covert and overt areas have been observed and reported and the observation section on Julie is now complete. It will help the staff identify those major areas of priority need satisfaction that can be tackled.

Julie is a good case for the observational process. Patients admitted to acute areas show obvious symptoms and inabilities, after all, that is why they have been admitted. But what of those already in hospital? The individual who has been in hospital for a considerable period of time faces a different set of problems. The influence of his environment, plus that of his condition, will be far more deep seated and he will have adapted to them so as to remain as anxiety-free as possible. In the majority of cases, this makes the observational element of the nursing process much easier to carry out, as there is a tremendous amount of background information. The nurse must ensure that she does not become confused by the patient's expectations of his hospitalisation and the institution's expectations of the patient.

READER EXERCISE

The example discussed above forms a good basis on which to establish observational skills, but each situation is bound to be different despite obvious similarities. Read the following case study and produce a suitable nursing impression and interview for a patient profile (Figs 3.4 and 3.5).

READER CASE STUDY: SUSAN

Susan is 18, unemployed and living at home with her parents. She is an only child. She is an outgoing gregarious girl who enjoys dancing, tennis, parties and going to discotheques. She has no steady boyfriend but does have a large circle of friends, all of her own age. Her parents dote on her and pander to her every whim. She is not short of money, but they are trying to encourage her to find a job. Recently she has been arguing with them quite often yet she indicates that she loves them both very much. Her parents describe her as a good daughter but a little childish at times. Since leaving school she has become a health food fanatic, eating only those foods reputed to enhance beauty and promote youthfulness. In the last 2 years she has lost nearly 30 kg in weight. She now weighs a mere 36 kg and is 5' 3" tall. Her mother says she will not eat at meals but picks at nuts and health food from time to time, and always follows these nibbles with a period of intense physical exertion, i.e. tennis, running, etc. When they have made her eat a meal they have heard her vomit in the bathroom shortly afterwards. She also states that much of her non-active time is spent in bed, something Susan never used to do. She has become forgetful of her personal hygiene and her father states that she has a strong smell of body odour about her.

ON ADMISSION

On admission she was rather over-active, and somewhat aggressive towards her parents. The social worker who accompanied them stated that they had argued all the way to the clinic. Susan's mother had to pack her case because Susan had stated she would not need any clean underwear. She said she only wanted to bring heavy jumpers and trousers despite the weather being exceedingly warm. Susan's vital signs were all normal except that she had a slight temperature. Routine urinalysis showed an increase in ketones.

INITIAL HOSPITALISATION

Susan has become solitary, refuses to eat anything at all and drinks only small amounts of water. She has lost a further 0.5 kg in weight and spends her time, when allowed, running everywhere. She has asked for a mirror in her room. She has not attended to her personal hygiene but has changed her clothes regularly though the soiled clothes are discarded without further thought. She has become abusive towards nursing staff who inhibit her physical exertions and refuses to see her parents who have visited twice. Her hair is lank and appears to be falling out by the handful. Her temperature is normal. Urinalysis still reads an increase in ketones.

SUMMARY

In this chapter, we have looked at what observation means to the psychiatric nurse and how it may be carried out. We have discussed the difference between observation and assessment, and have devised a system which will enable us systematically to correlate our data. The combi-nation of nurse's impression and interview gives to the nursing team a clear picture of the presentation displayed by the patient; each has its own advantages and covers different aspects of the profile. The requirement for the observational tool to be adaptable has been shown to be of paramount importance. Observing what is happening to the patient and what he feels about it provides the nurse with the basis for her care plans, as it is from here that we move to the nursing assessment and diagnosis.

REFERENCES

Abdullah F 1957 Methods of establishing covert aspects of nursing problems. Nursing Research 6: I: 4–23

Abdullah F, Martin A, Beland I L 1960 Patient centered approaches to nursing. Macmillan, New York

Bunch E H 1985 Therapeutic communication: is it possible for psychiatric nurses to engage in this on an acute psychiatric ward? In: Altschul A T (ed) Psychiatric nursing. Churchill Livingstone, Edinburgh

Elder E 1978 Transactional analysis in health care. Addison Wesley, Menlo Park, California

Geitgey D A 1969 Self pacing. A guide to nursing care. Nursing Outlook 17(3): 48–49

Henderson V 1960 The nature of nursing. Macmillan, New York

Jukes M 1987 Assessing the whole person. Senior Nurse 6(3): 14–16

Kron T 1981 The management of patient care. Putting leadership skills into practice, 5th edn. Saunders, Philadelphia

Marriner A (ed) 1979 The nursing process: a scientific approach to care. C V Mosby, St Louis, Ch 2

Miller A 1984 The nursing process and patient care. Nursing Times 80(8): 56–58

Peplau H E 1960 Talking with patients. American Journal of Nursing 60: 964–966

Peterson E A 1987 How to meet your client's spiritual needs. Journal of Psychosocial Nursing 25(5): 34–39

Roper N, Logan W W, Tierney A J 1981 Learning to use the process of nursing. Churchill Livingstone, Edinburgh

Smith L 1980 A nursing history and data sheet. Nursing Times Psychiatry under review 76(17): 18–23

Williams M A 1960 The patient profile. Nursing Research 9: 122–124

SUGGESTED READING

Cosmides L 1989 The logic of social exchange. Cognition 31(3): 187–276

Fox M J 1971 Talking with patients who can't answer. American Journal of Nursing 71(7): 1146–1149

Kessler A R 1977 Pitfalls to avoid in interviewing patients. Nursing US 7(9): 70–73

Topf M 1988 Verbal interpersonal responses. Journal of Psychosocial Nursing 26(7): 8–16

Your turn—question of the month: What do you need to know about patients on admission to manage their behaviour safely? 1989 Journal of Psychosocial Nursing and Mental Health Services 27(12): 32–33

Progress Notes

Nursing impression

Full name: _Julie Dawson_   Name preference: _Julie_

Clinical area: _Bowthorpe Villa_   Hospital number: _40790_

Observational period: _21.5.91 — 25.5.91_   Nurse's signature: _A. Sleigh_

Information source: _Patient, Mother, Social Worker, G.P., Visiting Psychiatrist, Ambulance Crew, Nursing Team, Admission Notes, Fluid, Sleep, Bowel Charts._

Date	
21.5.91	_Patient_ : Solitary, uncommunicative, preferring to remain in her bed away from contact with others. Refuses to sleep, eat regularly or take fluids. Does not attend to washing herself, or take interest in keeping her clothes clean. Seems indifferent towards staff, though 'blesses' them regularly. Behaviour is constant, becoming progressively more disturbed ie appears to have auditory hallucinations which are more noticeable when she is left alone. Seems to have taken solace in the bible — most conversations having religious overtones. Poor concentration. Seems most satisfied when discussing religion. Mother visits regularly (twice daily) although no obvious contact is made — Does not discuss visits.
	Mother : States she has never been like this before. Has always been interested in religion, but never taken it particularly seriously.
	Social Worker : States bedroom at home is extremely untidy — dirty washing everywhere, with scraps of food hidden under the bed, pillows and wardrobe. Discovered sheets of paper with mystical and religious writings on them with particular reference made both to Julie and her work-mates.
24.5.91	_G.P._ : Felt she was incapable of leading an independent life being totally dependent on her parents.
	Visiting Psychiatrist : Felt Julie was not capable of leading a satisfying existence within her own home. No real contact with her own environment.
	Ambulance Crew : Said she had no idea where she was.
	Nursing Team : All find it difficult to relate to her. No one has established any relationship with her. Only seems to be interested in them whilst talking about religion or related topics. Needs prompting to maintain her own basic functions.

Fig. 3.2A Julie Dawson's nursing impression.

Progress Notes Continuation

Date	
	Admission Notes: These reflect a downward trend in her ability to relate to her environment. She is doing even less for herself now than when she was admitted, particularly personal hygiene, eating, sleeping, drinking and interacting with those around her.
26.5.91	_Clinical Charts:_ These show that she is constipated, her skin condition is deteriorating, has had only 8 hours sleep since admission, seems less communicative in the company of more than one other person. Will only discuss topics related to religion.

Fig. 3.2B   Julie Dawson's nursing impression (cont'd).

Nurse's Interview

Full name: *Julie Dawson*   Name preference: *Julie*

Clinical area: *Bowthorpe Villa*   Hospital number: *40790*

Interview date(s): *24.5.91 25.5.91 27.5.91*   Nurse's signature: *Stephp*

Interview

Item ① *Attention to Activities of Daily Living*

response '*I don't have to wash anymore — God keeps me clean*
'*Sleeping is for the weak*'
'*I can only eat food which has been blessed' and if
I don't eat there is no need for me to go to the toilet.
I have eaten food that wasn't blessed, that is why I
have this stomach ache!*'
'*I will be told by him (pointing upwards) what I need to
do for myself.*'

Item ② *Her Awareness of her Surroundings and their Implications*

response '*This is my chapel, only those who come here will have
eternal life and I must bless them.*'
'*I don't understand why people keep coming in and out
and asking me if I am 'ok! It is them we must worry
about — I am very well Thank you!*'
'*I would prefer it if I could be left alone with my thoughts*'.
'*Only in this room (Her own bedroom) can I be truly happy.*'

Item ③ *How does she experience her own condition*

response '*I am in no pain, and I will only be happy when everyone
has been to see me! I am lucky to have God to talk to me.
I don't need to talk to anyone else so I don't need
to read or write anymore. Peace will come to me when
my mission is complete!*'

Item ④ '*What would she like the staff to do for her*'

response '*What staff, do you mean the angels? You must help
me to do, what God asks of me and keep my earthly
body as he desires it!*'
'*Help me to carry out my mission.*'

Fig. 3.3A Julie Dawson's nurse's interview.

Side two

Item

response

Item

response

Item

response

General impression of patient during interview(s)

Very quiet and would not face me when talking. Her replies are constant, but she is not really sure of herself, always fiddling with her hair. Almost impossible to maintain conversation. Very hallucinated. No concentration. Smells of body odour.

Fig. 3.3B Julie Dawson's nurse's interview (cont'd).

Progress Notes

Nursing impression

Full Name: _____   Name preference: _____

Clinical area: _____   Hospital number: _____

Observational period: _____   Nurse's signature: _____

Information source: _____

Date	

Fig. 3.4A   Reader exercise: Susan's nursing impression.

Progress Notes Continuation

Date	

Fig. 3.4B Reader exercise: Susan's nursing impression (cont'd).

Nurse's Interview

Full Name: _____   Name preference:_____

Clinical area:_____   Hospital number: _____

Interview date(s):_____   Nurse's signature: _____

Interview:

Item
response

Item
response

Item
response

Item
response

Item
response

Fig. 3.5A   Reader exercise: Susan's nurse's interview.   © Longman Group UK Limited 1992

Side two

Item
response

Item
response

Item
response

Item
response

Item
response

General impression of patient during interview(s)

Fig. 3.5B Reader exercise: Susan's nurse's interview (cont'd).

4

Assessment

INTRODUCTION

In the previous chapter, we discussed a method of gaining a considerable amount of relevant information about a patient's level of function and activity. This is called, observation. The nursing observation is carried out so that the nurse can gain a behavioural profile of the patient. This profile holds the clues to the patient's specific requirements and, ultimately, it is from these clues that the nurse will determine the appropriate nursing intervention. This requires that the profile be assessed; assessment links the two elements of observation and care planning within the nursing process framework.

WHAT IS ASSESSMENT?

The word, 'assessment', is often used to describe a method of valuation, but here it is used in the context of measurement and comparison. Assessment is: the measurement of the patient's ability to function independently and the comparison of that ability with the level of behaviour he must achieve to bring about true self-sufficiency.

When this analysis is complete there may well be a deficit discovered in certain areas of function between the patient's actual behaviour and his optimal level of behaviour. This difference is translated into a statement of need on behalf of the patient. This statement is called the 'nursing diagnosis'. Thus, if we combine the observational activity with that of assessment, the nursing function is seen to be as shown in Figure 4.1.

The actual purpose of assessment is thus to establish from the profile just what it is that the patient cannot do for himself. It should be remembered that the nurse is trying to promote self-sufficiency, or at the very least some element of independence, so that the assessment should not simply be one of ascertaining what the nurse can do for the patient, but more what they can do together. Without accurate observation and correct assessment of the behavioural presentation, the patient's planned care will probably only reinforce and exaggerate the symptoms that he experiences.

For example, a nurse may, from her observations, assess a patient as having motivational problems because he refuses to dress himself, and therefore construct an intricate re-motivational programme. She may then discover that the patient feels he is going to be sent home if he shows that he is competent at carrying out a task for himself. Her intervention has thus served only to increase the patient's experienced anxiety levels, and the result of this may well be that he develops behavioural deficiencies in other areas. Thus, a patient correctly observed but incorrectly assessed will, through inappropriate nursing intervention, present a picture of total dependence in self-maintaining areas within a very short period of time; i.e. he will fail to wash, feed and eliminate of his own accord and will gradually become uncommunicative, hostile and suspicious towards the nursing staff. Eventually, he may adopt bizarre and antisocial behaviour in an attempt to gain the security he so desperately wants. This whole situation can be averted if a more enlightened approach to his assessment is carried out, one which involves:

- realistic assessment criteria
- the patient's total involvement in the assessment phase (Burgess & Burns 1990).

REALISTIC ASSESSMENT CRITERIA

The criteria for assessment must give the nurse a workable guide to human behaviour and its motivation which will enable her accurately to identify how best she may assist the patient. Several considerations must be taken into account:

- the nurse's understanding of the patient's requirements in relation to scientific understanding of human behaviour
- human needs theory
- the establishment of need priorities
- the recognition of
  — primary problems
  — secondary problems
- the patient's experience of his own needs/problems.

HUMAN NEEDS THEORY

In 1943 the American neo-behaviourist C. L. Hull postulated that all organisms' behaviour was designed to reduce needs, whether directly or indirectly. It should be noted here, however, that views on the underlying motivation of human behaviour differ. Thus, the five major schools of thought in psychology believe that human behaviour is motivated in the following ways:

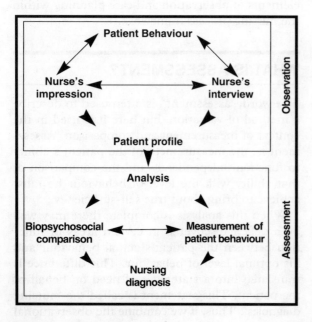

Fig. 4.1 Nursing function.

- psychoanalytical — unresolved childhood problems
- biological — body chemical activity
- humanistic — free will
- behavioural — learned stimulus/response
- cognitive — selective reasoning.

The principle of total need reduction is thus much disputed, in particular by the humanistic psychologists who believe in the total autonomy of the individual. However, the nursing process uses a diluted form of needs theory as the basis for its activity.

Human needs can be classified in several ways, but may be considered firstly in terms of their origin, whether they are:

- inborn
- partially inborn
- learned

and secondly in terms of whether their satisfaction is essential to the survival of:

- the individual
- the species
- the society in which we live.

Need satisfaction and human behaviour

If an individual fails to satisfy one of his needs, three basic courses of action are open to him:

1. He becomes frustrated, anxious, angry and irrational and develops aggressive behaviour to obtain what he needs.
2. He remains unsatisfied and anxious, possibly becoming resentful, irritable and uncomfortable. This failure will influence future behaviour connected with the same need, though not necessarily in an overtly aggressive fashion.
3. If the need is a basic biological one and it remains unsatisfied, he will die.

Need satisfaction, though not necessarily the only motivation for human behaviour, certainly constitutes a major part of human activity. A need only becomes a problem when it is not satisfied and it becomes a nursing problem when the indi-

vidual is not capable of satisfying it for himself. If the nurse is to recognise needs in her patients she must first understand their influence on her own life routines. Crow (1980) points out that needs' satisfaction is essential to both well and ill people: 'The only difference being that in health we can meet these needs for ourselves, but when ill we are dependent upon others helping us meet our needs.'

The work of Abraham Maslow has provided us with considerable information about human needs and is used here as an assessment model. In *A Theory of Human Motivation* (1943), Maslow isolated the factors he felt were responsible for human activity. He listed them in terms of priority, showing basic physical needs as those which the individual had to satisfy in order to survive, and others, such as aesthetic needs, as those which he would always strive to satisfy. Maslow felt that certain higher order activities, such as gaining personal autonomy, spiritual goals and self-fulfilment, were motivated by success with lower level needs. In nursing we are concerned with those needs further down Maslow's hierarchy, as their successful satisfaction should enable the individual to achieve understanding of his ability and potential. Other authors (Hertzberg 1968) have followed a similar path to that of Maslow; Evans (1980) used Maslow as a guide to patient needs and Kraegal (1972) also adapted his work to produce a patient need nomenclature (Fig. 4.2).

HOW TO ESTABLISH NEED PRIORITIES

Each person has evolved as an independent entity; however, because as human beings we have similar environments, social settings and biological predispositions, our needs too are similar, albeit to varying degrees. Therefore, if the nurse has an understanding of human requirements she should be able to identify areas of inability and incapability that affect her patient's behaviour. By being aware of an established hierarchy of needs, she should also be able to establish priorities for helping to satisfy those needs identified as being unresolved and, consequently, constituting a problem for the patient. She will

7 Aesthetic needs–Self-actualization
The need to realise your own potential and achieve personal autonomy. The need for order, privacy, beauty, truth and spiritual goals.

6 Cognitive needs
The needs for knowledge and understanding, comprehension and exploration, sensory stimulation, environmental and personal mastery.

5 Creative needs
The need for self-expression, production, creativity and usefulness.

4 Esteem needs
The need for dignity, respect, self-esteem, individuality, sexual identity, personal identity, recognition and deserved praise.

3 Belongingness and love needs
The needs for security, love, affection and companionship. The need to affiliate and communicate.

2 Safety needs
The need to be free from fear or threat of injury. The need to be able to depend on someone and to orientate oneself.

1 Physiological needs
The need for fluid, food, shelter, comfort, oxygen–to eliminate waste products of metabolism, sensory function, exercise and rest.

Fig. 4.2 An adaptation of Maslow's hierarchy of needs.

know that basic physiological needs must be dealt with first otherwise the patient will die. But she also knows that the patient is biopsychosocial and that the satisfaction of psychosocial needs are just as vital to the individual's well-being. The nurse may decide to attempt to help the patient satisfy

these needs in conjunction with the physical ones, or leave them until a later date; this will depend on:

- the individual's potential and capability
- the time available to her
- the resources available to her.

She will also know that if the individual is helped to satisfy his own physiological needs he will achieve both an element of dignity and personal identity which will in effect initiate the process of satisfying psychosocial or psychocultural needs.

The satisfaction of those needs on levels 5, 6 and 7 of Maslow's hierarchy (Fig. 4.2) comes through the individual's own experience and successful satisfaction of the initial needs, and consequently they are self-motivating (Catherman 1990). The nurse does not have the ability to help the patient with these areas on a direct basis. However, she is able, through her skills and professional training, to help the individual satisfy those needs on levels 1, 2, 3 and 4. The nurse must therefore concentrate on:

1. physiological needs
2. safety needs
3. belongingness and love needs
4. esteem needs.

Let us consider how this might take effect in an assessment.

Example 1

A patient is observed to be not eating at mealtimes and losing weight, having initial insomnia till at least 0300 hours, and failing to mix with any of his fellow patients. He has no visitors to the ward and will not initiate conversation with the nursing staff. He appears anxious and tense whilst in the company of others and refuses any form of communal therapy. Social skills' ability appears limited, as when in conversation his contributions seem hesitant and insecure, and he lacks self-confidence. His personal problems are totally unresolved as they are undisclosed due to his failure in real forms of communication. He states that he would rather leave hospital as he feels uncomfortable, and that he is sure he is wasting everyone's time.

The nurse identifies the following needs as being unsatisfied and therefore constituting a problem for him:

- Biological — eating, resting/sleeping, routine, sensory function.
- Psychosocial — communication, affiliation, freedom from fear, security, companionship, personal identity.

In terms of priority, she realises that he must satisfy his need to eat and rest as these are basic needs for sustaining his life, but she also realises that if he only eats small amounts he will not necessarily be in any real danger especially if he gradually increases his food intake as his appetite returns. Next, she identifies that satisfaction of the need to communicate represents the most important psychosocial element missing in his presentation. She knows that when she and the patient later decide on the approaches they can adopt to help in this area, she may well be able to deal with the other needs remaining unsatisfied in the psychosocial sphere, thus effectively reducing the amount of active nursing intervention required.

She therefore concludes that her patient's need priorities are:

- sleep/rest
- communication
- food.

It will be seen from this example that the nurse is not simply placing all the unsatisfied needs she identifies in order of procedure, but she is able to decide which needs she may reasonably not attend to, so that the satisfaction of the more important needs becomes more effective. In other words, the nurse is beginning to make herself more efficient and pertinent without losing the personal qualities essential for her to carry out her care. Another interesting fact in this example is that not all the unsatisfied biological needs identified are regarded as being 'top' priority. As long as there is a definite systematic approach to the assessment of observational material this situation may often occur, and nurses must be discouraged from always seeing the 'biological man' as the most important one.

Example 2

Paul, an acutely disturbed young man, is observed to be weeping whenever he is not in the public gaze. He is known to be experiencing both auditory perceptional disturbance and active delusional activity, and has serious thought disorders in the form of thought blocking. He has no insight into his condition and does not seem totally able to orient himself to his current geographical and sociological setting. Despite his psychiatric symptomatology, he remains spontaneous and even cheerful on approach, and almost completely independent in most activities of daily living. It has been noted that he requires minimal assistance in locating areas around the ward, i.e. kitchen and toilet, etc. He states that he is afraid, apprehensive and 'on edge' but cannot explain why. The content of his disturbance is unknown as yet, but obviously affects him in a very frightening fashion. He seems to be most at ease whilst sitting quietly in the nursing station with a member of the nursing staff, usually a male.

The nurse identifies the following needs as being unsatisfied and therefore constituting a problem for him:

- Biological — comfort, rest
- Psychosocial — freedom from fear, companionship, security, orientation.

In terms of priority the nurse recognises that the comfort and rest required by Paul will only occur when he is feeling safe, so she decides that the biological needs will be satisfied by her activity in the psychosocial area. She knows that he is afraid when left alone, and although she does not know the exact nature of his perceptional and cognitive disturbance she concludes that it must be contributing to this situation. She observes that he is most at ease in the company of someone that he perceives to be a 'safe' person, perhaps masculine, strong and confident; and she realises that the key to his presentation is his attempt to gain personal strength from other individuals.

Paul must become fully oriented to allow him to avoid the discomfort, pain and unpredictability of his self-made world, and this can only be done in the company of another 'real' person. She therefore concludes that her patient's need priorities are:

- orientation
- companionship.

Here, the biological component is regarded as a secondary consideration to the psychosocial elements. In a practical situation, it seems that nurses find difficulty in considering the psychosocial component first and often only physical problems are identified or, at best, are the only ones which receive intervention. The nurse must visualise the patient as a total entity and not simply as a chemical equation.

On the whole, it seems that the spiritual aspects of life, which constitute personal identity, are poorly interpreted by nursing personnel; and Sampson (1982) has highlighted the necessity of establishing patient needs beyond those recognised within the constricting medical approach if total patient/nurse intervention is to take place. Quality nursing care can only be achieved if the nurse is aware of the totality of her patient and is capable of systematically assessing his individual requirements at that given moment in time when she has been asked for help. It will also be noted from both the above examples that the nurse, in placing priorities on the satisfaction of certain needs, relegated others to secondary status. This is essential if full consideration is to be given to those elements of care delivery regarded as the key to patient independence. Sometimes, however, one problem may have the potential to cause another. The nurse has to be able to differentiate between actual and potential problems (Sanger et al 1988, Mulhearn 1989).

PRIMARY PROBLEMS

Keane (1981) stated that problems could be categorised as actual, potential or possible. If a person has one definite need which is not being satisfied it creates an actual problem. If this is not dealt with, it will lead to other, more involved problems, developing (potential problems). These in turn may cause other problems (possible problems) to arise at a later stage, although not necessarily, as it depends entirely on the

actual make-up of the individual involved. For example, if a young mother is admitted suffering from depression following childbirth, she has a problem with the depression affecting her ability to look after herself and maintain her own life. Potential problems that may result because of this are weight loss, constipation and toxic confusional symptoms. She may develop reinforced patterns of anti-social behaviour, or suffer social isolation and physical difficulties through anti-depressant and anti-psychotic medication. She may even attempt suicide. The result of these problems may well be that her husband leaves her, taking their child with him; she becomes ostracised by her family and the child has to be fostered. Ultimately, she will be unable to form a relationship with her own child, who may, as a result, develop a faulty personality, and all as the consequence of a few months' maladaptive behaviour.

Primary problems are actual problems – those needs that the patient is having difficulty in satisfying at the moment of intervention. They are often apparent to the observer but in a psychiatric setting are very rarely apparent to the individuals themselves. If they are accurately assessed and dealt with before they lead on to entrenched modes of maladaptive behaviour, secondary (potential and possible) problems can be averted. Unfortunately, in many instances, primary problems set up a chain reaction which is difficult to interrupt; often, the most the nurse can hope to achieve is to be aware of the possibilities and to slow down the sequence of events.

SECONDARY PROBLEMS

It is preferable to consider possible and potential problems under the heading of secondary problems. These are far more difficult for the nurse to assess. They will depend greatly on influences over which she has little or no control, i.e. social settings, family relationships and psychosocial make-up. Biological secondary problems are easier to identify because the nurse should be able to foresee these in the light of her knowledge of drug side-effects, treatment consequences and illness characteristics. When assessing observed information, the prediction of secondary problems occurring will depend entirely on the accurate appraisal of the patient's current life situation in relation to the following factors:

- the accuracy of the nurse's primary problem statement
- the complete treatment programme including the effects of nursing intervention
- the patient's personal relationships, both before and after the crisis
- the patient's personality, including motivational and spiritual concepts
- the pre-admission social and cultural setting and the changes that may have taken place within it
- financial and employment aspects
- speed of onset and prognosis of condition
- the patient's awareness of his present behaviour in contrast to his own evaluation of himself
- the patient's expectations of his hospitalisation and recovery.

However, although many of these factors are variable and may or may not have a direct bearing on the development of secondary problems, the patient's awareness of his own present behaviour and his resultant expectations will always influence the eventual sequence. It is, therefore, imperative that the nurse involve the patient in establishing the nature of current problems. In this way, the degree of personal responsibility required to promote recovery and independence can be initiated from the very onset of the nursing intervention.

PATIENT'S UNDERSTANDING OF HIS OWN NEEDS/PROBLEMS

If the observation section of the process has been carried out correctly, that is with the full involvement of the patient, then he will already be aware of the nature of the nurse's activities. The nurse will have discussed with him the rationale behind her activities so that, unless he is extremely disturbed, or his memory impaired, he should be able to relate this element of the process to what has gone before. He will be aware that the information gathered was specifically designed to gain a clear picture of his own requirements, so it must follow that he is expecting some kind of outcome from the initial activity.

The nurse must take her findings to the patient for his appraisal of the situation before she makes a final decision as to the best course of action to adopt on his behalf. Patients are often very surprised to find that the nurse is prepared to ask their opinion of what they think should happen to them, and what they think their basic problems are. They are even more surprised to find that, having given their opinion, the nurse actually discusses it with them and then comes to an agreement with them about how best to deal with the problems.

The patient must be offered an outline of the nurse's findings from the observation section and asked what he feels are the fundamental problems contained within it. This can be offered to the patient in the form of 'if you observed a man doing the following what sort of conclusions would you draw from it' or, 'what would you say was the problem, if you observed, as I did, the following situation'. In this way, the patient sees himself through someone else's eyes, in addition to the subjective viewpoint he has of himself. He is going to protect this subjective view of himself, no matter how distorted it might be, so it is vital that the nurse be as tactful and understanding in her approach as possible.

It is obvious that the nurse will already have begun to establish patterns and ideas prior to this meeting, but she must not be rigid in her beliefs about the patient, otherwise he will become aware that his opinion does not really matter. He will feel that she is only being polite. This can in itself reduce an already low self-esteem to a non-existent one and do untold harm to the rapport of mutual trust and acceptance that is developing through the nurse's close contact with him. In many cases, the patient will see things differently to the nurse, accepting one item as a problem, but not another. She must try to be as flexible in her understanding of the situation as possible and create a setting of mutual understanding and cooperation. It is important that the patient is not forced into participating against his wishes. The nurse must offer him various alternatives and if he refuses to take any of them, or chooses not to participate, this is his right. The nurse must allow the patient to exercise this right and find a more flexible approach to involving him (Waterworth & Lukes 1990, Hicks 1990).

The patient may have a different viewpoint about the priority of his problems, and the nurse must realise that he still expects something to be done about them or feels that he should be offered help to contend with them. If he does not receive that help he will feel cheated, resentful and unimportant. These feelings of frustration will be directed partly at himself but mostly towards the hospital staff and, in particular, the nurse. If, however, the nurse is prepared to look at his problems with a degree of sympathy which allows her to pin her understanding of his situation on the patient's reflected perceptional framework, far more will be achieved from the implementation of the necessary nursing intervention that follows because the patient feels more involved in his own care. We all have a need to feel that what we are doing is important and has value. It is one of our basic identity needs to feel that we have some control over what happens to us and to the things that go on around us. If the nurse denies the satisfaction of this need to her patient through the thoughtless way in which she provides him with the opportunity of setting his own nursing priorities, she has probably done more harm than good by her actions. What chance has the patient of achieving independence if the very vehicle through which it is offered inhibits his need for personal identity?

It is not suggested that the patient totally dictate his own priorities and ultimately his own nursing care. If he were able to carry out that procedure successfully, and without help, there would be no reason for his hospitalisation or for professional intervention. What is suggested is a joint project which might be carried out as follows:

1. The nurse highlights the major elements in her observed material.
2. She asks the patient for his opinion of his own needs.
3. They both discuss his ideas fully.
4. She outlines her own ideas and her impression of his needs.
5. They discuss any similarities or differences that occur in their separate assessments.
6. They agree on the best selection and priorities in relation to both assessments.

THE NURSING DIAGNOSIS

Until now the assessment of the patient's situation has been described as being due to either unsatisfied needs or problems, but these are unsatisfactory terms because they fail to give a true picture of what is taking place. They must be converted into terminology which describes the behaviour creating the health problem, in relation to its cause. This is called the 'nursing diagnosis'. It is a statement or conclusion about an observed pattern of behaviour presented by the patient. Definitions of the nursing diagnosis range from Abdullah et al's (1960) 'determination of the nature and extent of nursing problems' to Greenwood's (1955) 'determination of a phenomenon by systematic inspection', and are in line with later authors such as Johnson (1984), Loomis (1988) and Townsend (1988). All outline the diagnosis activity as being more than just a personal opinion or a wise judgement. Having looked at the knowledge base from which the assessment is made, those factors inherent in the diagnosis which renders it scientific as opposed to instinctive must be considered.

1. The nursing diagnosis is a descriptive statement. If the statement also contains the cause of the problem, aetiologically based, it has far more relevance to both patient and nurse alike.
2. It may, at times, be identical to the medical diagnosis; but two people with the same medical diagnosis may have a different nursing diagnosis, and two people with differing medical diagnoses may have the same nursing diagnosis. It all depends on the individual's response to his illness.
3. As it is a reflection of current patient behaviour, the nursing diagnosis differs from the medical diagnosis in that the medical assessment

remains the same throughout the whole illness phase, whereas the nursing diagnoses, changing as the patient's response to his problems changes, plots the progress of the individual through his own disability.

4. It is revised, through the evaluation of procedure, throughout the whole of the individual's contact with the nursing services.

5. The diagnosis statement must be clear, precise and recognisable, whilst corresponding to current terminology used within the discipline.

6. It must be as specific as possible so that there can be no doubt in the minds of those who read it as to what it means. It is totally inadequate to write one-word nursing diagnosis statements, as this will produce one-word objectives and one-word care provisions.

7. The diagnosis must come into effect as soon as the patient enters hospital, or comes into contact with the psychiatric nursing services, and it only ceases to be required when:
— The patient solves his problems and therefore does not need nursing care.
— The patient is discharged from the care of either the hospital/clinic or its supporting nursing services.
— The patient dies, in which case care will in part be transferred to the relatives until they no longer require the nurse's help.

8. A preliminary nursing diagnosis is required for a patient on admission, as it is necessary to initiate care from the very beginning of his hospitalisation. This type of diagnosis is called a tick-off diagnosis because as more is known about the individual so the assessment statements will become more specific as alternatives are ticked-off from the initial list.

9. If the decision to make a diagnosis is delayed for the purpose of collecting more data, this does not necessarily mean that the end result will be a better diagnosis. Someone once pointed out that the first idea a person has about a subject is usually a poor one. If he thinks about the subject a little more and gathers some more information he will have a much better idea. The best idea, however, never comes, so there must be a cut-off point, when you have arrived at a reasonable solution. The nurse has to accept that

she is not always going to be absolutely perfect in her appraisal of a situation.

The nursing diagnosis is thus as systematic and scientific as its medical equivalent. It is arrived at in exactly the same way, by carefully establishing a pattern of behaviour that when professionally reviewed produces data consistent with a known maladaptive response. The medical diagnosis will be a disease statement; the nursing diagnosis will usually be a behavioural statement which arises as a result of the medical one, although it must be said that there are occasions when they have no connections at all (Gordon 1987). Through careful examination, a patient's psychiatrist may diagnose the individual as suffering from a toxic confusional state. The nursing diagnosis will tend to centre around the cause of this condition and the resultant behaviour it produces. Take, for example, the case of constipation arising through low roughage content in diet, lack of physical exercise or a failure to answer the call to stool because of perceptional or memory impairment or even delusional activity. Here, constipation is deemed to be the cause of the condition; the aetiological factors of the constipation are considered so that a more specific nursing intervention can be devised.

NURSING DIAGNOSIS TERMINOLOGY

It has already been stated that the nursing diagnosis must be specific, contain aetiological features where possible and be precise. The following are examples of how a nursing diagnosis might be expressed:

- Failure to express himself in conversation due to lack of self-confidence.
- Initial insomnia till 2.00 a.m. due to anxiety related to his marital problems.
- Urinary incontinence throughout the day due to lack of geographical orientation.
- Inability to dress himself as he cannot clasp small items (buttons, etc.).
- Failure to communicate verbally because of prominent depressive features.

- Limited diet taken because of psychomotor overactivity.
- Verbally aggressive in the company of strangers because he fears their intentions.
- Poor personal hygiene because he cannot remember whether he has washed/bathed or not.
- Will not see his visitors because he feels ashamed of being in a psychiatric hospital.
- Experiences physical discomfort whilst sitting upright due to tender pressure area on right buttock.

These nursing diagnoses are descriptions of physical, psychological and sociological behavioural patterns and in themselves contain considerable information about what is happening and why, for anyone who reads them. As has already been said, they are statements relating an unsatisfied need to the behaviour that this lack of satisfaction has produced. For example, in the first item, the needs isolated are those of personal expression and identity, communication and affiliation, freedom from fear and the ability to depend on someone. It may not always be possible to be totally complete in the statement, especially when producing a 'tick-off' diagnosis, but it should always be the aim of the nurse to be as close to the principle of accuracy as the situation and information permit.

When constructing the diagnosis, it must be remembered that the patient will have been involved and will have access to the statements that the nurse documents. It is therefore essential that the following are always achieved:

- The statements are factual and not conjectural.
- The statements do not conflict with the patient's interpretation of conversations held with the nurse.
- There are no derogatory comments that deprive the individual of the dignity he deserves.
- Nothing appears on the documentation that has not been discussed at length with the patient.

It may be necessary to produce a statement which is only partially descriptive of the aetiology as it may be important for the patient to establish that aetiology for himself. Here, it is important that through exploration the patient, not the nurse, achieves satisfaction of his own needs, using the experience as a reward for his endeavour (Townsend 1988). The nurse's reward will come when the patient has been successful through her guidance. If, as is often the case with acutely disturbed patients, the patient totally rejects the conclusions and diagnoses of the nurse, the need for him to achieve some degree of equanimity, or come to some form of compromise, may itself be classified as a nursing diagnosis before anything else can be accepted. It must be said, however, that patients are far more prepared to compromise if they can see that they are working with the nurse and not simply being dictated to by her. This is where the mutual recognition of problems that take place during the nursing process has definite advantages over any other form of health care delivery system available to psychiatric personnel.

Before the case study, demonstrating the nursing diagnosis, the following aspects must be considered:

- How should the assessment for the nursing diagnosis be carried out?
- Who should carry it out?
- When should it be carried out?

HOW SHOULD THE ASSESSMENT BE CARRIED OUT?

The actual diagnosis must be made in collaboration with both the patient and other members of the nursing team. There should be a very definite procedure for the nurse who is carrying out the assessment to follow, on the lines of the flow chart shown in Figure 4.3.

The following guidelines should be observed if the activity is to be successful for both patients and staff.

1. The ward staff must agree on criteria for assessment which should be followed in all cases. Only by having these criteria can the nurse in charge of the team be expected to establish some

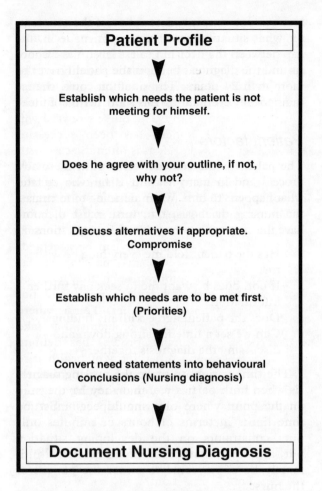

Patient Profile

▼

Establish which needs the patient is not meeting for himself.

▼

Does he agree with your outline, if not, why not?

▼

Discuss alternatives if appropriate. Compromise

▼

Establish which needs are to be met first. (Priorities)

▼

Convert need statements into behavioural conclusions (Nursing diagnosis)

▼

Document Nursing Diagnosis

Fig. 4.3   Nursing diagnosis flow chart.

degree of continuity amongst all those grades of staff qualified to make assessments.

2. Consultation with the patient must be maintained at a consistently high level so that total communication can be achieved. Much research has been carried out looking at the effects of communication on such areas as perceived pain, individual prognosis and treatment effectiveness. All studies confirm that the more the patient knows about what is happening to him, and why, the more capable he will become in dealing with a problem.

It is, in effect, removing the doubt in his mind which aids his progress. The element of doubt and uncertainty must be removed when his own nursing care is being discussed with him. If

throughout both the observational and assessment sections he is totally involved, then doubt, suspicion and anxiety can be minimised, thus enabling him to achieve the most from his encounter with the nurse.

3. Comparisons between other patients (and their respective nursing diagnoses) and the patient being assessed are counterproductive and inappropriate. In the long run they will produce stereotyped care which denies the quality of individualisation.

4. If a patient is assessed as having many different nursing diagnoses, only five of these should be used to provide the basis of care. Those remaining must be documented in the progress notes for future attention. If more than five are used, the quality of the care provided may suffer and the purpose and function of the diagnoses in the patient's care may become too confusing and difficult for him to assimilate.

WHO SHOULD CARRY OUT THE ASSESSMENT?

As has already been said, the assessment is a collaborative one between the patient and the nursing team. However, the final decision for the actual nursing diagnosis rests with the nurse who is carrying out the assessment with the patient. Ideally, this should be the same nurse who carried out the construction of the patient profile, as she will have a far greater insight into the patient's activities. Both the observation and assessment sections of the nursing process are a means to an end: the objective is for the nurse to gain a better understanding of the patient through the establishment of a solid patient/nurse relationship so that she can provide pertinent nursing care for that individual. It therefore follows that if Nurse Jackson constructed the patient profile it would be wasteful if Nurse Wilson replaced her to do the assessment. Much time would be lost filling in the personal gaps that would be left out of the clinical documentation, and considerable patient trust and confidence in the effectiveness and genuineness of the nursing team as a whole would be diminished.

It must be appreciated, however, that this ideal

situation is not always attainable because of sickness, shift changes, etc., so an alternative system must be available. If a junior member of staff is carrying out the assessment, she should use a member of the trained or senior staff as her guide. If the junior member is not available for the assessment, the senior member should be able to carry out the activity in her place. Likewise, if a senior or trained member of staff is carrying out the assessment she should use a junior or learner as if they were in a teaching situation. In the senior member's absence, the junior member can carry out the assessment under the guidance of another senior member of the team. In this way, both senior and junior staff will have their own case load and will be responsible to other members of staff for either guidance, teaching or back-up support for a further group of patients. As pointed out in Chapter 3, it is not appropriate to have untrained staff responsible for the production of the patient profile and the same applies to the assessment. Untrained staff have a definite commitment in both sections but this involves being a support system to the nurse, to whom they should direct all their information and observations.

WHEN IS THE ASSESSMENT MADE?

The time at which the diagnosis is made will depend on the situation being assessed and the patient with whom it is being carried out.

Admission factors

These will centre around the following:

1. whether the patient has been directly admitted or transferred, in which case the care provided may have to be changed from a traditional approach to the nursing process
2. whether this is a preliminary or tick-off diagnosis, or one of a continuous nature.

In both cases it is essential that the time between the information being gathered and the diagnosis being made is as short as possible. The tick-off diagnosis may be made within the first half hour of admission, although in some extreme cases it may be as soon as the patient

arrives. One simple rule to follow is that, no matter what situation the diagnosis is made in, the gap between the decision to establish the diagnosis and the diagnosis being made should never be more than 24 hours. The situation could change dramatically even during this short period of time.

Patient factors

The patient is the constant element in the whole process and in many ways it is he who dictates what happens to him. When deciding to formulate the nursing diagnosis, the nurse must therefore have the correct answers to these four questions:

1. Has the patient told me everything he wishes to?
2. If not, does he want me to seek any further information?
3. Does the patient agree with my findings?
4. Can we set a time for sitting down and discussing the diagnosis together?

The time is right to make the nursing diagnosis when both parties feel that they have agreed on the point where care should begin. Setting time limits in terms of hours or minutes only puts constraints on the developing situation but, as already stated, too much delay will ultimately be of no value to either the patient or the nurse.

DOCUMENTATION

The nursing diagnosis is recorded on the care plan (Ch. 5). Here, we will simply try to establish the flow that exists between observing behaviour and its assessment. Nurses should get used to the idea of writing down their findings whenever the opportunity arises. In psychiatry, the habit of personal notebooks does not seem as popular as in general medicine, but if the nurse is to make an accurate assessment of her findings it is essential that she puts them down on paper. When the assessment phase has been reached it is advisable that the information be sifted, the areas of need isolated and noted, a priority set and the whole thus converted to the various nursing diagnoses. The nurse has a far better chance of being accurate if throughout the whole procedure she makes notes which she can refer back to, and use as a visual aid.

SETTING PRIORITIES

In an ideal world, the nurse would be able to carry out an assessment programme, identify any number of different problems and convert them to nursing diagnoses. However, with as many as 10 patients in each care team or care group it would be pointless to produce long lists of problems that, from a purely logistical standpoint, could never be attended to. It is therefore necessary for the nurse to establish priorities when deciding what is to appear on the care plan. Obviously there has to be consultation with the patient and other members of the team but in the end it is the primary nurse who decides which nursing diagnosis is used.

Often, this form of prioritisation will help to define more clearly those areas which the patient finds particularly difficult to cope with. It is possible, too, that by dealing with these major problems some of the smaller ones may also be rectified. However, prioritisation is also important in helping to ensure that what is written on the care plan is what will happen. Thus, if only one problem can be dealt with for each of the 10 patients within a care group, there is little point in writing two or three per patient. If too many problems appear on the collective set of care plans for a care group the likelihood is that nothing will get done at all, or else that it will all be done one day, and nothing the next when there are not enough staff on duty. The resultant loss of continuity may have serious effects on the patient's confidence in the nursing team and on their ability to help him.

This process of refining and prioritising might be regarded as the 'lowest care denominator'. In other words what appears on the care plans is the absolute minimum that must be dealt with even if the worst possible staffing scenario is considered. Problems that cannot be dealt with immediately have to be put on hold until such time as the

opportunity arises to do so. The increase in continuity that arises from these actions should mean that more serious problems are offered more clinical time and are therefore likely to be dealt with more effectively. On the days when staffing levels are better, nurses should resist the temptation to start adding to the care plans until they are absolutely sure that they can indeed do what they propose.

In this book a maximum of five nursing diagnoses are used for each of the example care plans. This is done to give the reader more scope to explore the care planning process. In practice, it is likely that fewer problems would appear on the care plans because there may be insufficient staff to deal with them.

Chapter 3 used Julie Dawson's case study to show how the observation element of the nursing process might be carried out. Those observations are used here to demonstrate how the nursing diagnoses may be concluded. As it would be impractical to reproduce all of the information once again, only an outline of the basic points from the patient profile are given here. The reader may find it necessary to refer back to the case study in Chapter 3 for more detailed information.

CASE STUDY: JULIE DAWSON

Julie was admitted having withdrawn completely from her work, social and family commitments. She was uncommunicative in the extreme, almost totally dependent on the nursing staff for self-maintenance activities and her psychiatric symptomatology blocked her ability to relate to her present environment in any shape or form.

MALADAPTIVE BEHAVIOUR OBSERVED IN JULIE'S PRESENTATION

1. *Biologically based*

   - Only seven hours sleep in five days
   - Smells of body odour
   - Not eating
   - Not drinking
   - Does not go to the toilet
   - Has a stomach ache

- Skin condition dry and breaking down in pressure areas
- Lies around all day without exercise.

2. *Psychosocially based*

- Cannot concentrate for long periods
- Will not communicate with staff or fellow patients (or visitors)
- Will not leave her room to explore the ward
- Does not seem to know where she is
- Can only relate to religious activities
- Will not accept her surroundings at face value.

3. *Biological needs not being satisfied*

- Sleep
- Personal hygiene
- Food
- Fluids
- Elimination of waste products
- Physical exercise
- Freedom from pain.

4. *Psychosocial needs not being satisfied*

- Orientation
- Companionship
- Self-expression
- Usefulness
- Communication.

(It might be argued that Julie was trying to satisfy her higher needs (cognitive and aesthetic) without first achieving satisfaction of needs further down the hierarchy. In effect, she was running away from her responsibilities to herself.)

NEED PRIORITIES

Immediate need priorities   *Interim diagnoses*

- Sleep: Fails to sleep for more than 1–2 hours per 24-hour period
- Companionship: Cannot relate her feelings to anyone in her environment
- Physical activity: Remains physically inactive and lacking in exercise.

On-going need priorities   *Nursing diagnoses*

- Companionship: Cannot relate her feelings to anyone in her environment
- Physical activity: Remains physically inactive and lacking in exercise
- Usefulness: Cannot see any purpose in her real existence as she has nothing to do
- Personal hygiene: Fails to wash, dress or groom herself
- Food/liquids: Cannot see the reason for eating or drinking.

Julie's needs' priorities will alter after her initial contact with the nursing staff, so in this case both the tick-off and eventual nursing diagnoses have been included to demonstrate how the two may differ following the preliminary delivery of nursing intervention. The nursing sequence for establishing the diagnoses remains the same in the two situations, i.e., the nurse first records what she sees, then what this means, and then her conclusions about its effect on Julie's ability to function independently.

READER EXERCISE

The following is an outline of the reader case study from Chapter 3. It is suggested that the reader refers back to the case study and, using the headings listed below, documents the respective nursing diagnoses.

READER CASE STUDY: SUSAN

Susan was admitted to hospital because of her considerable weight loss and her inability to see the need to rest. She is resentful of her parents and because of her distorted body image has become aggressive and abusive towards the nursing staff who are trying to attend to her. She has no comprehension of the physical condition she is in, and her appearance is gradually deteriorating.

MALADAPTIVE BEHAVIOUR NOTED IN SUSAN'S PRESENTATION

1. Biologically based

2. Psychosocially based

3. Biological needs not being satisfied

4. Psychosocial needs not being satisfied

Need priorities   Nursing diagnoses

SUMMARY

In this chapter it has been shown that assessment is the comparison of an existing mode of behaviour with a desired one. A method has been chosen of establishing criteria for assessment – based on a modification of the human needs theory – which are then translated into the nursing diagnosis statement.

Throughout, a definite link has been established between the nursing activity outlined in this chapter and the patient's involvement in the whole process. It is understood that the reality of any clinical situation will dictate how far this principle can be carried out, but it must be appreciated that the more the patient can be made to feel that he should take part in the procedure which will eventually outline his treatment and nursing care, the more committed to it he will be. Ultimately, that commitment may be the one factor that decides whether a patient has a successful period of hospitalisation leading to personal satisfaction, or an unsuccessful hospitalisation leading to feelings or personal failure and frustration. Thus, while the nursing diagnosis is the goal of assessment, the means by which it is achieved is in many respects of far greater importance.

REFERENCES

Abdullah F G et al 1960 Patient centred approaches to nursing. Macmillan, New York

Burgess A C, Burns J 1990 Partners in care: patients as consumers of health care. American Journal of Nursing 90(6): 73–75

Catherman A 1990 Biopsychosocial nursing assessment: a way to enhance care plans. Journal of Psychosocial Nursing and Mental Health Services 28(6): 31–33

Crow J 1980 The effects of preparation on problem solving. Royal College of Nursing, London

Evans P J 1980 Thinking of Maslow. Nursing Times 76(4): 163–165

Gordon M 1987 Nursing diagnosis: process application. McGraw Hill, New York

Greenwood B 1955 Social science and social work. A theory of their relationship. Social Science Review 29: 20–33

Hertzberg F 1968 Work and nature of man. Staples Press, St Albans

Hicks B F 1990 Respect: a part of caring. Imprint 37(2): 43

Hull C L 1943 Principles of behaviour. Appleton-Century-Crofts, New York

Johnson M N 1984 Theoretical basis for nursing diagnosis in mental health nursing. Issues in Mental Health Nursing 6: 53–71

Keane P 1981 The nursing process in a psychiatric context. Nursing Times 77(28): 1223–1224

Kraegal J M et al 1972 A system of patient care based on patient needs. Nursing Outlook 20(4): 257–264

Loomis M E 1988 Discussion: psychosocial nursing diagnosis. Archives of Psychiatric Nursing 2(6): 357–359

Maslow A H 1943 A theory of human motivation. Psychological Review 50: 370–376

Mulhearn S 1989 The nursing process: improving psychiatric admission assessment. Journal of Advanced Nursing 14: 808–814

Sampson C 1982 The neglected ethic: religious and cultural factors in the care of patients. McGraw-Hill, New York

Sanger E, Thomas M D, Whitney J D 1988 A guide for nursing assessment of the psychiatric in-patient. Archives of Psychiatric Nursing 2(6): 334–338

Townsend M 1988 Nursing diagnosis in psychiatric nursing. F. A. Davis Co, Philadelphia

Waterworth S, Luker K A 1990 Reluctant collaborators: do patients want to be involved in decisions concerning care? Journal of Advanced Nursing 15(8): 971–976

SUGGESTED READING

Berthot B D, Lapierre E D 1989 What does it mean: a new scale for rating patient behaviour. Journal of Psychosocial Nursing and Mental Health Services 27(10): 25–28

Bryant S O, Kopeski L M 1986 Psychiatric nursing assessment of the eating disorder client. Topics in Clinical Nursing 8(1): 57–66

Essex B, Gosling H 1982 Programme for identification and management of mental health problems. Tropical Health

Series, WHO. Churchill Livingstone, Edinburgh

McBride A B 1990 Psychiatric nursing in the 1990's. Archives of Psychiatric Nursing 4(1): 21–28

Thomas M D, Sanger E, Whitney J D 1986 Nursing diagnosis of depression: clinical identification on an in-patient unit. Journal of Psychosocial Nursing and Mental Health Services 24(8): 6–12

5

Setting objectives

INTRODUCTION

The subject of this chapter represents the very essence of psychiatric nursing as it is known today and forms the medium through which it can grow for the future.

When a potter takes a piece of clay and places it on his wheel, he has in his mind's eye an idea of how he will shape it, so that it becomes an object of worth and admiration. He shapes and moulds the clay with the skill and dexterity that only a craftsman can achieve, and when he has finished he has fashioned a unique object, despite its resemblance to any other he has manufactured before. Some people call this skill art, others simply creativity or talent, but however it is described, it is satisfying and worthwhile for the potter and those who admire the object long after he has completed his work.

The setting of objectives is the point in the nursing process where the nurse can begin to use her skill and dexterity in the same way as the potter, except that here the clay is of the human kind. By taking her assessment of the patient and formulating in her mind's eye a picture of what she hopes to achieve then manufacturing a method by which she hopes to reach that goal, she is introducing an artistic quality into her work that offers both her and her patients the opportunity of achieving unique possibilities. This stage is called 'planning nursing care'.

Of course, the analogy between the nurse and the potter is not strictly appropriate. The nurse must combine her scientific knowledge of her subject matter with a creative approach to her end product, acting always within the strict confines of that original knowledge. It is not the intention here to enter into a lengthy discussion as to whether nursing is an art or a science; but it must be remembered that if a subject is approached in too scientific a manner it becomes cold and clinical, while if it is approached from a purely artistic viewpoint it becomes far too subjective and unpredictable. Nursing is a creative activity carried out within a scientific framework.

SETTING OBJECTIVES

An objective or goal within the nursing process is a statement concerning the expected outcome of nursing intervention. Once written, it tells the nurse what it is she is hoping to achieve with her patient. More importantly, it is a method of communicating intent, not just to patient and nurse but to any other health care representative involved in the programme. It is constructed from information described in the nursing diagnosis. If the diagnosis is taken as being the negative aspect of the patient's behaviour, then the purpose of the nursing intervention must be to create a positive one and this purpose is stated in the objective. The following factors form the basis of an objectives construction:

1. It should describe the patients behaviour.
2. It may be either behavioural or expressive in nature.
3. Only one objective should accompany each nursing diagnosis, unless they are written in a sequence.
4. It should always be patient centred.
5. It should be easily attainable.
6. It should be provable.
7. It may be quantitative.
8. It must be precise.
9. It should contain a time limit.
10. It should be a positive statement as opposed to a negative one.

EXPECTED PATIENT BEHAVIOUR

If the nursing diagnosis describes the patient as having difficulty in relating to other people, the objective must state how he will relate to people after the nursing care specifically designed to help him in that problem has been given. For example; the patient will remain calm in the company of others; he will look them in the face; he will remain in their company; he will initiate conversation; he will think about what is happening to him when others try to talk to him. These statements are all positive ones, i.e. they say what the patient will do. Nurses should avoid using negative statements, such as: he will not shout at them; he will not walk away from them. Positive statements imply that the patient is learning to use more effective personal strategies, whilst negative ones imply that he is simply not to use old and ineffective ones. One offers alternatives, the other highlights failure.

BEHAVIOURAL OBJECTIVES

Objectives are goals or targets designed to give individuals a sense of direction for their actions. We set objectives for ourselves in all sorts of situations. If we are booked to go on holiday, we work out how much money to save each month so that we will be able to pay for it. If we do not save enough, we do not go on holiday. To save the required sum is an objective. When we wake in the morning we decide upon things we want to do during the course of the day, then spend the rest of the day trying to get all those things done. These too are objectives. If a patient decides that he will gain a certain amount of weight, or improve his personal hygiene in some way, or discuss his problems with his primary nurse, or even decide not to speak to people who annoy him, these too are objectives. The examples quoted above are all of a particular type of objective called behavioural objectives, because they describe a mode of action or behaviour that the individual must carry out.

To fully understand the nature of objectives, it is necessary to explore the context in which they arise. If we use the example of the holiday once again, the purpose of the saving is to have the satisfaction of going on holiday, which in turn provides us with all sorts of different types of satisfactory experiences. The holiday itself is not the reason for saving, more the benefits that the holiday brings. These may include the need for change, rest or excitement, exploration, enjoyment or fun. These benefits constitute the overall objective and the monthly savings are the individual objectives set to eventually achieve that aim. Each objective requires us to do something, i.e. put money in the bank, thus describing a happening, or an event or behaviour. The proof of this behaviour is the increase in the balance of our bank account. If the money increases, then by definition the behaviour must have been carried out. As will be seen, not all objectives function in this way and therefore not all can be measured using the same process, but in the case of a behavioural objective, the performance of an act or the carrying out of a task or action or some other observable activity is always necessary for it to be achieved.

Behavioural objectives are often the first type that nurses learn to use because they tend to be easier to understand and construct. They are particularly appropriate for patient care, or patient activity, whenever some form of observable behaviour is required. They are probably most effective within the biological and sociological domains, where success is usually gauged by the use of demonstrative acts.

The main positive attributes of behavioural objectives include the following:

1. They are prescriptive — they outline the rules by which they are to be achieved.
2. They specify an outcome — the end product is clearly defined.
3. They specify exact options — the circumstances surrounding the activities are carefully controlled.
4. They are suitable for behavioural change — behaviour within the physical and social domains are most accessible to these objectives.
5. They identify a mode of action — they describe exactly how an activity should be carried out.

Behavioural objectives are not always the most suitable form of objective as some behaviours are far less demonstrable or observable than others. In certain circumstances such objectives may actually be counter-productive. The main negative attributes of behavioural objectives include the following:

1. They do not offer free choice — the patient is not at liberty to choose the nature of his eventual presentation. In most cases it is often a question of achieving or not achieving.
2. They do not allow for diversification — changes are not made according to spontaneous requirements. As behaviour is absolute there can be no half measures.
3. They are dedicated to baseline behaviours — there is always a level regarded as the optimum performance. This is measured in terms of improvement/decline.
4. They are rarely multi-dimensional — alternative approaches are seldom available, with the result that care becomes stereotyped.
5. Only the obvious problems are dealt with — because the alternatives are limited, the patient's potential for real problem-tackling is not exploited.

Great care must be taken when using behavioural objectives that the traps listed above are not fallen into. Nurses should be as critical of their statements of objectives as they are when evaluating their own clinical performance. Should they find themselves producing objectives which seem ineffective or unrewarding, then it may well be that they have chosen to use the wrong type. If the patient appears unhappy with the direction of his care, or expresses dissatisfaction with his progress, or simply does not respond to the demands of problem-tackling, these too are indicators that a different form of objective may be required.

EXPRESSIVE OBJECTIVES

Strictly speaking, expressive objectives are also behavioural, because of course all human actions involve some degree of action or response. The main difference lies in the degree of behaviour and its intention. With behavioural objectives, the behaviour itself is the desired response; but with expressive objectives, it is the significance to the patient of individual and personal experiences which are far more relevant. This type of objective concerns itself with the thought processes behind the behaviour, and strives to give the patient some understanding of why he feels and behaves the way he does. Inherent in this approach is the belief that if the patient attains a greater level of self-awareness then he is in a better position to alter his responses by choice rather than simply as a result of demands placed upon him by others. Thus, expressive objectives are central to the development by the patient of real problem-tackling, because their main thrust is basically intellectual and emotional (Ward 1989).

The expressive objective is designed as a medium through which themes can be developed, skills and understanding expanded and elaborated, problem-tackling facilitated, and diversity encouraged. Sometimes referred to as 'experiential' objectives, they encourage the patient to explore and make sense of his own feelings. More significantly, they do not demand that set behaviours are the outcome of their usage but, rather, that the patient becomes more aware of himself. The only demand placed upon the patient is that he initiate the process; the response is purely of his own choosing. For example, after asking a person to think about how he feels when someone appears to reject him, it would be pointless to tell him that he feels rejected. He may say that he does not really feel anything at all, and that if the person does not like him then that person has every right to reject him. He may say that he feels angry and hurt and would like to strike out at the person responsible, or he may say that he feels cold and lonely and probably deserves to be rejected because he is so totally useless. All of these responses are different, yet all are 'correct' because they are pertinent to the individual who experiences them. The nurse cannot dictate the outcome of an expressive objective and therefore they become more the responsibility of the patient.

The vast majority of psychiatric patients experience emotional or intellectual difficulties with which only expressive objectives are really equipped to deal; thus, the psychological and sociological domains are often the best areas for their usage. Moreover, psychiatric problems do not readily conform to the unilateral demands placed upon them by the rigid observational nature of the behavioural objective, so it is vital that expressive objectives are used whenever the opportunity arises.

Nearly all intellectual activities in which a patient might be involved are legitimate targets for expressive objectives. Areas such as self-awareness, esteem activities, assertiveness and problem tackling, counselling, personal identity routines and the psychosocial aspects of the more traditional behavioural therapies, such as relaxation and social skills training, all lend themselves to the flexibility and personal nature of expressive objectives. The difficulties associated with dramatic psychological disturbance – always resistant to any form of behavioural objective because the latter require that the patient use memory and comparison at a time when these are least accessible to him – are another obvious area for the expressive form. The elderly, with their acute memory difficulties, have less trouble responding to questions about their feelings than they do about locating the lavatory, whilst an individual undergoing prolonged and sometimes apparently endless social rehabilitation would benefit greatly from some appreciation of his psychological ordeal.

Expressive objectives are statements which include words such as 'explore', 'think', 'consider', 'look at', 'compare', 'analyse', 'use', 'contrast', 'imagine', etc., and contain phrases such as 'put yourself in the place of', 'imagine you are', 'what happened before you', 'how did you feel when', 'what are you trying to do when', etc. All of us use expressive objectives in our daily lives. When something happens to us, we often find ourselves reflecting upon it later in the day in an attempt to make sense of it, or to decide upon a better course of action or simply to remember it. When someone else tries to give us advice on the matter, we may feel that their advice is inappropriate to us, but that decision is made on the basis that we have already started to make sense of it all for ourselves. Our objective was to 'sort things out in our own mind'. In effect, that is just what an expressive objective is all about.

The main positive attributes of expressive objectives include the following:

1. They are evocative—the patient examines his own memories and feelings rather than dealing with rules set down by the nurse.

2. They do not specify an outcome—no targets are set, just that the patient consider the problem in his own way.

3. They describe a personal encounter—no procedures or routines are involved, as the patient chooses his own way of doing things.

4. They allow free choice—the nurse cannot dictate outcomes or conclusions.

5. They are suitable for personal development—the scope for greater self-awareness enhances the patient's potential for personal growth because he is not hampered by behavioural boundaries.

6. They are most suitable for psychosocial difficulties—because of the intellectual nature of the expressive objective, they enable the patient to tackle problems by analysing their feelings rather than altering their responses to them.

It is the element of patient autonomy inherent within expressive objectives that makes them such a useful planning tool when dealing with problems that require the patient to take responsibility for his own decision-making processes. Change takes place because the patient decides that this is necessary and not, as with the behavioural model, because a response is identified by others as being unsatisfactory. For this reason, not all problems can be dealt with using expressive objectives, because not all problems are of such a fundamentally intellectual nature. However, as so much of the expression of mental ill health centres around emotions, relationships and communications, the nurse must try to use experiential objectives if some real internalised changes are to be made in patient behaviour. A patient who always verbally abuses female nursing staff must be given the opportunity to consider why he does it, what effect it has on others, what he hopes to achieve by it, if he can achieve these things in another way, if he is happy with what he is trying to do, if there are other more complicated reasons for choosing women to abuse, how he looks in the eyes of others when he behaves like this, and what alternatives are open to him, rather than simply being told to 'Stop it', as if he were some small child being naughty in the school playground. The expressive objective offers dignity and equanimity in such circumstances because it does not deny the patient his own feelings.

Expressive objectives are not as easy to formulate as their behavioural counterparts because they demand a higher degree of tolerance on the part of the nursing team, and they require nurses to be more analytical of their patients behaviour. It is much easier for a nurse to say to a patient, 'Don't do that, do this', than it is to say, 'Explore your feelings about female nurses and then we will sit down and discuss them'.

The negative attributes of expressive objectives include the following:

1. They are difficult to construct—a much greater understanding of the patient is required before they can be formulated, though they may be used in information gathering routines.

2. They are unsuitable for biological problems—they may be used as a complementary part of the care programme to explore the emotional side of physical problems, but not for the problem itself.

3. They require the patient's cooperation—because so much is required of the patient, without their support the expressive objective becomes unusable.

4. They can exacerbate a problem—if a patient is confronted with real elements of personal incompetence, he may elect to increase his helplessness rather than adapt to it.

5. They demand intense nursing support—on a practical level, it may not be possible to spend enough time with a patient once the exploratory work has begun.

SELECTING THE APPROPRIATE OBJECTIVE FORM

It is important, particularly within psychiatry, that nurses use the most appropriate form of objective for the patient's needs. Depending upon the presentation of the patient's problem, the parameters set by all those involved and the eventual expectations that the patient has, nurses need to establish which is the most suitable form at that moment in time.

There is no set pattern to the choice of objective. The same problem may be presented by two separate patients on the ward and require different objectives, one behavioural the other expressive. In most cases, patient's care plans contain a combination of the two types of objectives, and in some instances an expressive objective may be written and linked to a behavioural one for the same nursing diagnosis. For example, a patient who refuses to look people in the eye when he is speaking to them might be expected to:

1.   consider the feelings that he has when he looks someone in the eye
2.   write down those feelings for discussion with his primary nurse later in the week.

It is important that nurses do not use a single objective form for all patients, nor select one particular problem as always requiring a particular type of objective. A creative, imaginative and exploratory approach to objective selection is called for, with the main criteria for selection being that which will offer the patient the most chance of personal success, reinforcement or reward. Ultimately, it is the patient who determines the effectiveness of objective selection, both at the time of inception and during its evaluation. Nurses should not be afraid to change the format if one particular form does not seem satisfactory. After all, we cannot expect our patients to explore new ideas if we are not prepared to do so ourselves.

Thus, combining objectives, using more than one type of objective for each nursing diagnosis with one complementing the other, altering the form if and when necessary, exploring alternative approaches for each nursing diagnosis and then communicating the rationale for all this work in a way that makes sense to the patient, are some of the skills required of the psychiatric nurse when developing action sequences for the construction of care objectives.

ONE DIAGNOSIS—ONE OBJECTIVE?

Wagner (1969) described setting an objective for each problem perceived as being one of the four essential components of a care plan. As it is suggested that a maximum of five problems appear on the care plan, it follows that five objectives will also be present on that care plan. However, this may not always be the case. In some situations, objectives for different nursing diagnoses will be similar, but it must be remembered that the objective is specifically designed for one patient so they will vary according to his present situation and condition, environment and potential for change, etc. The nurse is trying to show how that patient will progress in each problem area, so the objective must be specific to that problem. Blanket statements for several problems such as, 'rehabilitate to community environment' have little meaning as far as nursing direction is concerned. Such situations may well occur, but only as a result of the interactive process of several other smaller and more specific care objectives having already been met. As the problem changes, so will the objective. As the degree of maladaptive behaviour is reduced, so the objectives will find new areas to explore for an increase in adaptive behaviour.

On some occasions, one nursing diagnosis may have both an expressive and a behavioural objective attached to it in an attempt to develop different themes with the same problem. Skilful use of objectives may also produce a situation where one nursing diagnosis produces a series of objectives, linked sequentially to produce an action sequence. Wagner's idea of one objective, one nursing diagnosis is still appropriate, but creative nurses should never be tied to regarding this as an absolute rule.

PATIENT ORIENTATION

All through this book it is emphasised that the process of nursing is a mutual activity involving both patient and nurse. Thus, when the objectives are set they should be agreeable to both parties. The patient has a good idea of his capabilities no matter how disturbed, disoriented or distressed he is. In many respects, he may actually dictate how the objectives are formulated. He is not likely to be motivated to succeed in areas he does not recognise as problems, or travel along care paths he feels are irrelevant. Sometimes it is necessary for the nurse to construct objectives knowing that they have little chance of success, to allow the patient the opportunity to experience the situation for himself; the use of expressive objectives can be invaluable at such times. The patient and the nurse should sit down together and discuss the objectives. Although the nurse should already have an idea of what she hopes to achieve, she should be prepared to adapt these ideas to the needs and wishes of the patient (Faulkner 1985, Teasdale 1987).

REALISTIC OBJECTIVES

It would be foolish of a nurse to write such a statement as 'gain 10 kg' as an objective for a newly admitted girl with severe weight loss problems just as it would be foolish to tell an alcoholic to stop drinking, or a fish not to get into water. It might take that girl many years before she manages to get her weight loss under control, and then only after she has gained an understanding of why it is happening; in some cases that is never. An objective must be a goal that can be achieved with some degree of ease, certainly at the beginning of care. The success of achieving initial goals builds up confidence and stimulates the potential for further successes. In some situations, therefore, the initial objectives must be virtual inevitabilities. For instance, if a man is admitted with severe restrictions in his life because he absolutely must carry out certain time-consuming yet irrelevant actions, his first objectives might be that he does not exceed a slightly longer period of time in the bath than that which he is already taking, or he is allowed extra attempts than he really requires in making and remaking his bed. The idea is that the patient is offered a degree of manoeuverability and not simply played into a corner and expected to make radical changes in entrenched behaviour within the first few days of his admission. It should be remembered that hospital admission usually

causes an increase in perceived anxiety levels, so in many cases the patient will appear to get worse rather than better during these first days. The objectives for care must take account of this. At a later stage in the care, the objectives can become more demanding, but then there will be a cushion of success behind the patient that will, in effect, act as a stimulant for greater achievements.

In many cases, patients appear to progress through their nursing care in a series of peaks and troughs. They will be successful in achieving their care objectives in a certain problem area for some time, and then get stuck and seem incapable of getting any further. At this point, the nurse has to be adaptable enough either to reduce the level of behaviour expected through care intervention, or to change the objectives altogether. The nurse's sensitivity in this particular area is essential if eventual success is ever to be gained. She must explain the situation fully to the patient as being a normal event, otherwise frustration and despair will take the place of success and satisfaction.

PROVABILITY

Question: How can a statement be proven?
Answer: In the case of a behavioural objective – if it can be seen. In the case of an expressive objective – if it has been attempted. (Expressive objectives are not validated in the strict sense of the word 'proven' – the proof is only that the patient made an attempt and even then the outcome cannot be regarded as either desirable or undesirable, for this is the patient's domain, not the nurse's.)

The way that objectives are made provable is by ensuring that their formulation contains verbs. Verbs are 'doing words' – they require an action to take place – and action can be observed or discussed afterwards. Often, nurses write aims as opposed to objectives and aims are too non-specific to be of value in care planning. The two elements necessary to ensure provability are:

1. that they should be as specific as possible, isolating exactly what area is to be worked on.

2. that they should contain action words which can be monitored in terms of patient activity for comparison against the original statement, or discussed at a predetermined later date.

How does this work in reality? Consider two objectives, one acceptable, the other not:

- Objective A: 'The patient will be less anxious'.
- Objective B: 'The patient will be able to sit and read a newspaper'.

Objective A is in fact an aim, and it is of no value because the only way by which it can be assessed as having taken place is a subjective one. Moreover, if the objective setting and evaluation are carried out by different nurses, how can the second nurse possibly have any idea of whether or not the patient is 'less anxious'.

Objective B is much better because the nurse has looked at the effect of anxiety and discussed with the patient a course of action that would be possible if he did not experience so much anxiety. It can be assessed by any nurse who observes the patient, simple questioning proving whether or not the paper has actually been read. The objective can therefore be proven, and, more importantly, can be done by any member of the nursing team.

In the same way, expressive objectives can be formulated so as to enable some degree of validation. Although in theory any expressive objective is 'provable' some formulations are less acceptable than others. For example, one would never write, 'Patient will consider the meaning of life', but might consider, 'Patient will consider his place in his family and discuss this with me at end of week 1'.

QUANTITATIVE STATEMENTS

We would not dream of going into a greengrocer's shop and asking for 'a few apples' or 'a couple of carrots'. Similarly, the nurse must not make statements such as, 'He will eat more today than yesterday', or 'He will sleep longer tonight than last night' as her objectives for the same reason:

they give no clue as to quantity. Quantitative elements are essential for the construction of behavioural objectives, though of less value for expressive ones. Quantitative objectives are far easier to evaluate and also to carry out, because both parties have an amount, level or percentage to aim at.

Take objective B once again. The behaviour required has already been stipulated but it must be made quantifiable if it is to become a more valuable statement. For example:

The patient will be able to sit down and read a newspaper for five minutes each day.

The inclusion of the words 'five minutes each day' tells all concerned how much behaviour is expected before the objective is reached. Such information as times, weights, strengths, etc., when written into the behavioural objective statement, provides the patient with a specific goal to aim at.

PRECISE STATEMENTS

If the objective is written in a verbose and lengthy way, nursing colleagues will pay little attention to it because to do so would be both time-consuming and boring. If nurses are not prepared even to read the elements of the care plan, they cannot produce the care necessary for the relief of the patient's problems. Objective B might look like this when prepared correctly:

Will read a newspaper five minutes per day.

Or, similarly,

Will write his feelings down and discuss them with me at 6 p.m. Friday evening.

Of course, it is possible to reduce the objective statement so dramatically that it conveys nothing at all to the nursing staff, i.e. 'continent', 'cheerful', 'relaxed', 'active'. One-word objectives will produce one-word care, which will be equally useless to patient and staff alike.

TIME LIMITS

The setting of time limits within the objective statement is necessary so that evaluation of the care provided can be carried out. It is good, sound practice to reward someone for their actions as soon as possible. If there is no time limitation within an objective, then successful actions will not receive their just rewards from the nursing staff in any formalised fashion and will therefore not reinforce the action for future progress. Time limits vary but can range from as little as 15 minutes in an acute situation to anything up to two weeks or more in more controlled and slower paced ones. A simple rule of thumb for deciding on time limits is to remember that, in most situations, the longer it takes to develop maladaptive behaviour the longer it will take to change it to adaptive behaviour. Objective B might look like this after the inclusion of a time limit:

In one week he will read a newspaper five minutes per day.

Or, similarly,

Will write his feelings down each evening and discuss them with me at 6 p.m. Friday evening.

It is important that the nurse does not set objectives that are to be evaluated months ahead and require very intricate behavioural changes, as the patient will lose sight of his target and become disinterested in his care. To avoid this, two different types of objectives which relate to different time spans must be used.

1. long-term objectives
2. short-term objectives.

The long-term objective is the eventual behavioural presentation anticipated by the nurse after anything up to a year's nursing intervention. The short-term objective is the behavioural presentation anticipated by the nurse after as little as two or three days of nursing activity. Altogether, there may be as many as 50 or 60 short-term objectives leading to the eventual achievement of the long-term objective. It is wrong to ask a patient to aim straight away at the long-term objective, because he will almost certainly give in or lose his way within a very short period of time.

OBJECTIVE SEQUENCE

The last consideration to be made concerning objectives is the way in which their sequence is formulated to produce the outcome described.

Consider the case of a man who has difficulty relating to others. He becomes noisy and verbally aggressive when approached and will not enter into a reasonable conversation with anyone. This situation has been developing for several years and, therefore, it will be extremely difficult to reverse the pattern. What follows is the possible objective sequence that may be followed for this man. The reader must bear in mind that each objective must be achieved before the next one is attempted, so in a real clinical situation you cannot produce this type of sequence at the beginning of care intervention: it develops as you progress. It may, of course, be possible to outline such a plan with a view to adapting it if it becomes unattainable.

Nursing diagnosis (see Fig. 5.1)

Becomes verbally aggressive when approached for conversation.

Patient care objective

1. After 1 week, will remain quiet in the company of a nurse sitting close by for 5 minutes.
2. After 1 week, will remain quiet in the company of a nurse sitting close by for 5 minutes morning/afternoon.
3. After 1 week, will remain quiet in the company of a nurse sitting close by for 1 minute per hour.
4. After 1 week, will remain quiet in the company of a nurse sitting next to him for 1 minute per hour.
5. After 1 week will remain quiet in the company of a nurse who greets him and sits beside him for 1 minute each hour.
6. After 1 week will remain quiet in the company of a nurse who greets him, asks one simple question and sits beside him for 1 minute each day.
7. After 1 week will remain quiet in the company of a nurse who sits beside him and makes small talk.

A sequence which uses expressive objectives might read like this:

1. The next time he becomes verbally aggressive the nurse will ask him to describe the way he feels.
2. The next time he becomes verbally aggressive he will try to explain why he feels the way he does.
3. After the next verbally aggressive incident he will try to put himself into the place of other people to see how he affects them.
4. He will list those things that happened to him before he became verbally aggressive. He will discuss these with the nurse at the end of the week.
5. He will keep a personal record of the times he felt like verbally abusing people, and why, and discuss this at the end of the week.
6. The nurse will spend a half hour each evening discussing the day's events and his behaviour towards others.

It is unlikely that either of these two sequences would be able to function without the other, so the nurse would probably compile a sequence incorporating features from both.

The above sequences are incomplete but will be built up so that eventually the long-term objective is achieved and the patient is able to build on his confidence and ability to communicate in a reasonable way, and feel safe and secure with the experience of his own success.

There are many variations to the sequences described, for example:

- the inclusion of other staff members
- varying the staff concerned
- using other disciplines – occupational therapists, psychologists, etc
- involving other patients
- slowing the sequence down by reducing the expected behaviour change
- extending the time limits
- speeding up the sequence by increasing the expected behaviour change
- reducing the time limits.

The permutations are limitless – but they are all planned. To summarise: objectives should have the following properties:

- specific
- quantitative (in the case of behavioural objectives)
- brief (or as brief as possible)
- timed
- sequential.

DOCUMENTATION

Objectives may be documented by the nurse made responsible for the patient's care, but under the guidance of the supervising nurse, sister or charge nurse. In some instances, senior ward staff may decide to write all the patient objectives themselves, but this should only be done in consultation with the appropriate junior staff who have already gathered and assessed the relevant patient information. Failure to do so could easily result in inappropriate objectives being constructed and lead to disasters in patient care. The long-term objectives are written in the patient's progress notes and cross referenced for easy access at a later date. This is necessary, as with the time factor involved, staff changes and medical treatment activities, it is important that all staff have access to the eventual outcome of care in the various problem areas. The short-term objectives are written on the patient's care plan, sometimes called a nursing analysis sheet or a nursing action sheet. As described before, this document also contains the relevant nursing diagnoses and, as will be seen, will also include the particular nursing interventions necessary for achieving the objectives. The care plan to be used is shown in Figure 5.1.

PATIENT CARE PLAN

As McCarthy (1981) stated, the care plan is actually the written transaction of the nursing process. Let us consider what Figure 5.1 contains:

1. *Identification.* Either the patient's name, clinical area or hospital number should head the sheet to ensure that the correct patients receive the care intended.

2. *Date.* This is the date when the nursing diagnosis is made and the care plan initiated. As the care progresses, it will represent the date at which new objectives are employed for the same diagnosis.

3. *Nursing diagnosis.* As many as 5 different diagnoses may be written into the plan, although this is an absolute maximum and nurses should try to restrict themselves to the number they are sure they will be able to deal with any one time.

4. *Patient care objectives.* These must be written at the same time as the diagnoses. They are numbered to correspond with the appropriate diagnosis for easy reference.

5. *Review date.* This date will be stipulated in the objective; some care plans do not have a separate area for the review. It is included here because it offers an easily identifiable reminder for evaluating patient care.

6. *Nursing intervention.* Again, this is numbered to correspond with the appropriate diagnosis and objective, thus giving a pattern to the plan.

Many care plans may be made out for the same patient during a long period of hospitalisation, so it is a good idea to number each sheet to maintain the sequence. They are stored in the nursing station or office with the patient's progress notes, so that a total picture may be gained of the patient's care and his response to it. In effect, the care plan states the problem, what is to be done about it and how it shall be achieved, while the progress notes act as a diary, recording what has taken place. All care plans must contain at least the following three items if they are going to be of any value:

1. the nursing diagnosis
2. the patient's care objectives
3. the nursing intervention, management or care.

Many also contain additional information, but it is important that the plan does not become a confusing document, otherwise nursing personnel will be unwilling and even unable to use it.

PATIENT INVOLVEMENT

Is the patient entitled to have access to his own care plan? The answer will depend on individual staff attitudes, hospital policy and the type of clinical area involved. In many cases the answer is 'yes', for the very reason that it is his plan. The more communication can be improved through written aids to which the patient can relate and refer the better. In some instances, patients discuss their care plans with their visitors and relations and involve them in their care planning. This should be the nature of the nursing process – to involve all those who have some concern with the patient – but it can be difficult to build this into the initial implementation of the system. If the patient is to be allowed access to his care plans, the way they are stored and the degree of availability must be carefully considered by the ward team.

Before discussing the type of nursing intervention to be employed, we return once more to the case study. The reader will see that the nursing diagnoses from Chapter 4 have been entered onto the care plan. In each case, where necessary, both the long-term and short-term objectives are isolated, with a brief explanation for them. In the clinical situation, documentation of the rationale for the objectives will not be necessary, as they will be discussed by the team and the patient.

CASE STUDY: JULIE DAWSON

Julie's short-term objectives – Patient Care Plan No. 1 (Fig. 5.2)

- Problem 1. Will achieve a sleep pattern with a minimum of six hours sleep.
- Problem 2. Will discuss her experiences of illness with the nursing staff.
- Problem 3. Will participate in all personal and ward-based routines.

Julie's long-term objectives – Patient Care Plan No. 2 (Fig. 5.3)

- Problem 2.⎫
- Problem 3.⎭ Unchanged
- Problem 4. Will write a letter to her parents.

Patient Care Plan

Patient name: ....   Clinical area: ....

Date	Nursing diagnosis	Patient/nursing objectives	Review date

Fig. 5.1A   Care plan.

Primary nurse:		Sheet number:	
Nursing interventions	Evaluation	Date	Nurse's initials

Fig. 5.1B Care plan (cont'd).

Patient Care Plan

Patient name: .Julie. Dawson............   Clinical area: .Banthorpe. Villa...........

Date	Nursing diagnosis	Patient/nursing objectives	Review date
26/6/91	① Does not sleep for more than 2 hours per 24 hour period.	① Will sleep for 3×2 hourly periods during a 24 hour period.	1/7/91
26/6/91	② Cannot relate her feelings to those around her – unable to establish a relationship.	② Will remember the name of her interviewing nurse and/or will say something of how she feels.	1/7/91
26/6/91	③ Remains physically inactive, sitting in her room all the time.	③ Will make a 1 minute excursion from her room every working hour.	1/7/91

Fig. 5.2   Julie Dawson's interim care plan.

- Problem 5. Will bath, dress and maintain herself on a daily basis.
- Problem 6. Will maintain body weight at lowest point on her weight chart whilst taking 2.5 litres of fluid per day.

The interim care plan and the on-going one have been separated to demonstrate the link between the two. In reality, the plan would be used until it no longer had any space left on it. Notice that each problem retains its own number on the two plans, with any new problems being assigned their own number. The objectives are numbered in accordance with their appropriate problem. (Note also that problem 2 has both an expressive and a behavioural objective with either being used as appropriate.) In this way a check can be kept on the number of problems encountered, and confusion is reduced to a minimum, as should a previously resolved problem reappear it is allocated its original number. The long-term objectives for Julie are written into her progress notes and will be referred to at each evaluation or review date. On Care Plan 2 (Fig. 5.3), the long-term objective of problem 1 has already been achieved so there is room for the inclusion of problem 6. In the case of problems 2 and 3, only the first short-term objectives in the chain have been achieved so their next stages

must be outlined. Only the right side of the care plans have been included here, the left sides appear in Chapters 6 and 8.

READER EXERCISE

State objectives for Susan here; and document your reasons for them (Fig. 5.4).

SUMMARY

Objectives in nursing terms are not offered as a 'cure' for the patient's ills but as an attempt to offer him the independence and dignity their achievement will produce. The nurse succeeds in her action if she helps her patient to do those simple things in life that everyone else seems to be capable of doing. When he has managed to carry out these activities he will be able to consider the difficulties which have denied him his self-sufficiency, and tackle them in the

Patient Care Plan

Patient name: ...Julie. Dawson.......... Clinical area: ..Bowthorpe. Villa.........

Date	Nursing diagnosis	Patient/nursing objectives	Review date
1/7/91	② Cannot relate her feelings to those around her — unable to establish a relationship.	② Will discuss her feelings with the allocated nurse at least once during each shift period.	8/7/91
1/7/91	③ Remains physically inactive, sitting in her room all the time.	③ Excursion time increased to 2 mins each, and also at meal times.	8/7/91
1/7/91	④ Cannot see any purpose in her real existence as she has nothing to do.	④ Will prepare a list of those things she sees others doing that she would like to do herself. Discuss with allocated nurse.	8/7/91
1/7/91	⑤ Fails to wash herself, dress or groom.	⑤ Will take a daily bath.	8/7/91
1/7/91	⑥ Cannot see the need to eat or drink.	⑥ Will remain in the dining area during meal times.	8/7/91

Fig. 5.3 Julie Dawson's on-going care plan.

knowledge that he does so as an independent person, not a social invalid. Nursing by objectives allows the nurse to place in perspective the care she provides and gives meaning and purpose to her actions. Objectives organise the nurse's approach to patient care. By enabling long-term objectives to be tackled in simple, easily attainable and realistic stages, the nurse produces the motivation and encouragement for success in both her patient and herself.

Patient Care Plan

Patient name: ....   Clinical area: ....

Date	Nursing diagnosis	Patient/nursing objectives	Review date

Fig. 5.4   Reader exercise: Susan's care plan.

REFERENCES

Faulkner A 1985 Nursing: a creative approach. Baillière Tindall, London

McCarthy M M 1981 The nursing process: application of current thinking in clinical problem solving. Journal of Advanced Nursing 6: 173–177

Teasdale A 1987 Partnership with patients? The Professional Nurse 2(12): 397–399

Wagner B M 1969 Care plans: right, reasonable and reachable. American Journal of Nursing 69(5): 986–990

Ward M F 1989 Expressive objectives. Nursing Times 85(51): 61–63

SUGGESTED READING

Clarke D 1990 Nursing: a problem-solving or a need-meeting activity? Senior Nurse 10(2): 13–14

McMahon R 1988 Who's afraid of nursing care plans. Nursing Times 84(29): 39–41

6

Care planning

INTRODUCTION

Having established via the objectives what it is that the nurse hopes to achieve within the care programme, the next step is to decide how these objectives are to be accomplished. This stage is variously known as nursing care, nursing prescription or nursing input, but we will refer to it here as nursing intervention. The intervention described on the care plan must be specifically designed to bring about the objective; this is the 'doing' stage of nursing. The planning of care must be approached scientifically. It is not acceptable for the nurse simply to write down the first thing that comes to mind. Various approaches need to be assessed, where possible offered to the patient for discussion, and a decision made as to which will offer the patient the best opportunity for success. Intervention activities must be well understood, or have a known outcome. It would not be appropriate to experiment with new models or strategies on the patient. Their effects could never be fully appreciated until after they had been used and this might cause alarm or concern for the patient for whom the outcome needs to be reasonably predictable. It is also important that a style of intervention found to be suitable for one patient is not automatically chosen for every other patient. Nursing intervention, like every other stage of the nursing process, must be selected and planned to suit each individual patient, and not the patient adapted to suit the intervention.

LINKING OBJECTIVES AND NURSING INTERVENTION

When planning intervention the nurse must ask herself the following questions:

1. Is the intervention appropriate to the objective?

This is established by looking at the intended outcome of the intervention and comparing it with the expectations of the patient's behaviour.

2. Is the care specific?

It is of no value writing intervention statements such as 'to reassure' or 'to support', for these are aims: they state what the nurse hopes to achieve, not how things are to be achieved. If the nurse intends to speak with the patient for a period of 5 minutes each hour so that she might help to develop interactive confidence, then this must be stated. Specific intervention statements might include:

- Will help patient grasp buttons on her blouse whilst dressing.
- Will act out a situation with him which happened during the day.
- Will sit with him without pressurising him to speak for one minute each hour.
- Will congratulate him for sitting with the other patients at meal times.
- Will discuss why he feels the way he does after his family have visited him.
- Will sit down and explore with him things that he feels have been important to him during the day.
- Will indicate the toilet sign to Hilda once every half-hour.

3. What is the best way of expressing the care I wish to give?

The proposed intervention is written down on the care plan in such a way that every one concerned, including any nurse allocated to work with the patient, knows exactly what is to happen. Nurses acting as key workers with a patient—i.e. someone who works specifically with a chosen patient or group of patients either because they require specific clinical input in an area where this nurse has recognised skill, or because they have a particularly effective relationship with the patient—will also need to ensure that the intense level at which they may be working is accurately communicated to nurses acting as relief during days off, etc.

4. Have I provided enough care?

One objective may require many different intervention statements which in turn demand actions at irregular intervals. The nurse must ensure that each one is documented, leaving none to be guessed at. Of course, the nurse must also resist the temptation of providing too many intervention statements, as this will overload the system; this will mean that interventions are only partially provided and have the knock-on effect of interfering with the interventions being offered to other patients. Care plans must be realistic if they are to be used.

5. Have I selected the best approach?

There are several ways that this can be decided. Marriner (1979) suggested using care conferences, in which the ideas, techniques and strategies used by individual nurses could be shared so that others might learn from them. Such conferences could happen at hand-overs, or be incorporated into evaluation sessions. In a community setting this would be more difficult, and some form of peer evaluation session would have to be formally convened (Ward & Bishop 1986). Other ways of carrying this out might include:

- Setting up peer review groups with senior nurses on a regular basis to consider a particular care programme for a patient once discharged.
- Case presentations, where a primary nurse discusses the approaches used by the team.
- Ward teaching sessions, in which either an

educationalist or one member of the nursing team passes on information about personal technology to nursing students.

- Allocating nursing students to skilled nurse practitioners so that specific clinical expertise can be considered. The evaluation of this activity would provide data about the intervention pattern.

It is of course important that junior members of the care team have access to the skills of the more senior staff, as otherwise no professional growth will take place.

6. Can the intervention be evaluated?

This question is perhaps more significant in the case of care offered for behavioural objectives, the expressive ones requiring no specific outcome except that the patients attempt them at their own chosen level. However, qualitative statements are far easier to evaluate, even in the case of expressive care. If the nurse stipulates times, amounts or degrees of intervention, and uses where and how statements, it requires only a simple cross check to establish if the intervention has indeed been offered in such a way. This can also be used as a method of evaluating the correct quantity of care being offered (Pesut 1989).

7. How will the patient react to the selected intervention?

The selection of interventions will almost always be that of the nurse, but this does not mean that the patient should have the care he receives sprung on him from out of the blue. The patient should be consulted wherever possible, and his likes, dislikes and preferences should always be a major consideration for a nurse who is planning intervention for a patient who does not wish to be involved. Even in such situations, before the final decisions are made the patient should have everything explained to him so that he understands the rationale for the proposed programme and the actual activities can be explored in detail so as to allay any confusion or concern. The patient may still be anxious about the intended nursing intervention, but at least he now knows what it will involve. Of course, individual responses to interventions will be as varied as the patients to whom they are offered, but if the nurse does everything possible to ensure that the patient's rights are respected and his wishes explored and acted upon, the dignity of the clinical environment will be maintained and any decision the patient makes about the intervention will be an informed one (Waterworth & Luker 1990).

CARE CONSIDERATION

The problem that exists in many psychiatric nurses' minds is that they cannot see the difference between the therapy they provide on their own initiative and the medical treatment prescribed by the doctor. It is not absolutely necessary to divorce the two because they should work in harmony, not antagonistically, but they still remain two very separate entities.

The major therapeutic component that nurses have to offer the patient, in his quest for independence, is their own personal expertise and the quality of the interactions that stem from it. The nurse does not prescribe medications or any other physical method of treatment, though of course she administers them and uses her knowledge to assess their suitability and effectiveness. What she does prescribe is perhaps far more fundamental to the well-being of the individual patient (Meades 1989). She offers herself as a counsellor, teacher and professional friend at the interface of interpersonal relationships. She is a mediator between what the patient can do and what he is capable of doing, and she acts as a stimulant to help him to realise these capabilities. In short, her main therapeutic tool is her own personality. When it comes to offering care she must write her personality clearly into the prescription. Time spent with the patient in planned activities is the only way she can ever hope to achieve the objectives she and he have set for themselves. There is no substitute for good nursing care to aid patient recovery, and this remains true despite the technological advances of the last twenty years.

When deciding on the types of intervention to be utilised, it is important to consider that all of them should contain the active element of the nurse herself or at least one of her representatives. One of the basic problems that exists for psychiatric patients, is their relationships with the world about them. It is the nurse's responsibility to adjust these relationships so that the patient can recognise them, understand them and eventually use them to gain the most from them. As stated previously, this constitutes the creative element within the scientific approach to nursing, because what happens between two people, no matter how planned, is always prone to spontaneity and improvisation. It is difficult to plan these things into a personal approach to another human being but that does not mean that the nurse does not try to use intervention which is open to this sensitivity. A little time spent examining alternative approaches to straightforward and often boring procedural approaches may well reap dividends far beyond the nurse's expectations. Sharing her ideas with her colleagues, seeking the advice and experience of her peers and passing on her perceptions of her own activities can be an exciting prospect for the creative nurse. She becomes the agent through which all intervention is offered, just as the patient becomes the centre around which all activity occurs. If one follows this philosophy, nursing care statements which do not include the nurse in some way, are seen to be a waste of time.

COMPUTER-AIDED CARE PLANNING (CACP)

The nurse has a responsibility to use all resources to improve the effectiveness of the care planning process, and this includes the use of computer technology.

In the early days of computer-aided care planning (CACP) very few individualised options were available to the nurse, and CACP could really only be used with standard care plans. Such systems were of great use in clinical areas with a fast turnover of patients, such as day-surgery, treatment clinics, etc, as they could save

the nurse a great deal of time. However, in areas such as psychiatry, the benefits of time-saving were more than negated by the resultant lack of flexibility. In addition, software packages which attempted to integrate care planning with nursing process activities and other managerial procedures were often far too difficult to use effectively, whilst those that required the nurse to undergo a considerable amount of training were often found to be unsatisfactory because the emphasis was placed more upon the needs of the manager than those of the clinical practitioner.

The actual technology used within these early systems was also somewhat uninspiring, with monochrome screens and very little in the way of user/computer interaction. However, the current generation of CACP systems have been designed primarily with the nurse in mind, in that:

1. The languages used by computer programmers have become space-efficient, so that computers can do more, but not at the expense of speed or ease of use.

2. Computer software companies have recognised that nurses need care systems which allow for flexibility and can be adapted to suit a variety of different client groups.

Software packages have in general become far more 'user-friendly', thus increasing the nurse's effectiveness. Nurses can now use CACP systems to produce a complete range of client/patient-centred strategies which cover a full range of nursing process activities and can be adapted to work with any number of different models of nursing. Although care must be taken in the choice of the software, CACP offers considerable advantages if used correctly.

ADVANTAGES OF CACP

The best care planning systems are those which have been developed with the needs of patients taking priority over other considerations. Such systems must be powerful enough to enable the nurse to interrogate the data that they contain concerning care planning activities, but also simple enough to be used by any of the clinical team no matter how limited their computer literacy.

Finally, they need to allow the nurse, or the manager, to extract information about any aspect of the care planning process so that more effective use of clinical resources can be achieved. Such a system has been developed by FIP (1991) and it is considered in detail below to examine the benefits such systems offer to the practising psychiatric nurse.

The FIP Care Planning System, was developed to meet the demands of practising nurses for a programme that would enable them to plan care using modern technology, but without losing the flexibility of traditional techniques. Although originally intended for use within a medical/surgical environment, the system is equally at home within a psychiatric one. It contains all the advantages one would expect from a fully integrated package. These include:

- Use of colour as a medium by which the nurse can tell which part of the programme is being used.
- User-friendly presentation.
- Fast amendment facilities.
- Standard, or core, care plans which, once set up, can be either used as they stand or edited to fit the needs of the individual patient.
- They enable the nurse to generate a totally new care plan for each patient.
- The ability to be connected up to other systems so that different wards and departments can talk to each other.
- The system runs via a user-defined nursing model.
- The stages of the nursing process constitute the action sections of the package, with problems, goals/outcomes, interventions and evaluations being used as the headings for each of the sections.
- Extensive user-created libraries of information from which the nurse can design individual or core care plans.
- Free text facility to cover ad hoc information which is not yet in the libraries.
- Security features which enable primary nurses to restrict access to client's care plans.
- Keyword search facilities so that a nurse looking in the library for a particular problem,

intervention or outcome statement can do so without having to type in whole sentences.
- Prompt facilities so that care is updated and evaluated according to pre-set times and dates.
- Printing facilities which enable the nurse to print out ad hoc, daily or episode care plans.

Nurses considering the use of a CACP package should compare the above facilities with those that their own system offers. If the nurse does not have the freedom to construct individualised care plans relatively rapidly and from an existing stock of pre-generated libraries, and if the system cannot utilise information about both nursing models and nursing process, the package is not suitable for use within a psychiatric setting.

USING A CACP SYSTEM

A suitable CACP system must also be easy to use. Again, the FIP system will be considered as an example of how such systems should work.

Stage one: library set-up

Perhaps the most time-consuming of all computer activities is the setting-up of the system. The nurse has to put into the computer's memory lists of problems, care outcomes, nursing interventions and evaluation statements; these are called *libraries*. Care must be taken at this time, for if the information stored is of poor quality, inaccurately written or too brief, then this will reduce the quality of the information that the nurse will ultimately get out of the computer when it is up-and-running. This library information can be collected by nurses working on the wards or in the community, by reviewing statements that have been made manually in the past. Some will appear on a regular basis, others only once, but the beauty of putting them into a computer library is that they can be stored and used as required, without the nurse having to re-write them each time.

The FIP system allows for different libraries to be set up, so you could have both a library containing those statements that are commonly used, and one that has those used less often.

When first using such a system, nurses often assume that they cannot feed statements into the computer because of the individualised nature of their work. However, a careful review of their care plans often reveals that in fact they often replicate statements for different clients, with perhaps only personalised components such as names, dates and amounts being changed each time. This is in effect what the nurse is going to do using the FIP system, only it will be written and edited much more quickly, especially if the initial libraries have been comprehensively constructed. The other great advantage of this system is that it encourages nurses to do this work, not outside agencies or even nurse managers. So this initial work stimulates nurses to question their own clinical actions and assess their current care planning performance.

Stage two: nursing model set-up

The second stage involves telling the computer which nursing model to use. FIP's system enables two models to be used at any one time. Any model can be used but, as it will determine how the patient's profile is constructed and ultimately prompt the nurse to gather information in a set way, time must again be spent getting the model into the computer properly. Most clinical areas will already have a working philosophy and be using a particular model of nursing. Before choosing to place this model in the computer, time should be spent evaluating whether the model has performed as intended and if it really is suitable for the area. This is therefore another review period, and decisions made at this time will affect the way that care is handled once the CACP system becomes active.

Stage three: operational use

Once the libraries and nursing model have been set up, the nurse can actually start to use all the information that has been fed into the computer and run the care planning programme. The FIP system is designed so that the need for keyboard skills in operational use is kept to a minimum.

This is achieved by the facility to move to the desired option on the screen using horizontal and vertical arrow keys, and to select the option using the 'enter' key. This system works in the following way:

1. The computer asks the nurse for her password; once given this allows access to different levels of the programme.

2. A menu screen asks if new patients are to be added to the existing list or if the nurse wishes to edit an existing patient's care.

3. If new patients are to be added, then the programme moves to the section dealing with the patient's profile and problems are identified using the model of nursing. The nurse either selects from the problems in the libraries or, if the problem is unique, enters a brand new one for this patient. In most cases the problems in the libraries are either appropriate, or there is one that is close enough to be edited for use with the new patient. Free text is available as a last resort.

4. The nurse then moves to the outcomes part of the programme, where again there will be a selection of objectives related to the specific problems that the nurse has already identified. As with the problems, if an outcome relevant to this patient is not in the libraries then it can be generated for him, though an existing one can be edited or personalised for him. Review times are placed on the individual outcomes and the nurse will be prompted by the computer when this time has arrived.

5. Nursing interventions are the next part of the programme; again, the nurse has a wide variety to choose from in the library, or specific ones can be constructed.

6. The programme is checked and saved. It is now ready to be printed out and used.

7. Evaluation of outcomes is carried out on the basis of whether or not the objective is achieved, and there is a space for the nurse to write a comment regarding the process.

8. The whole care programme for the patient can be viewed, adjusted, edited or completely re-written according to the changes in the patient's health status.

The printed copy of the care plan is used by the nurse in exactly the same way as the handwritten type, except that (1) it has taken much less time to prepare and (2) because it has been printed and not handwritten, there is less chance of it being misread or misinterpreted. Of course it may not be necessary for the nurse to print the care plan as it may be sufficient to use the screen copy. This saves yet more time and increases confidentiality. Nurses from the individual teams wishing to see what is on their patients' care plans merely call them up on the computer, view them and then allow the programme to return to the opening screen once again, ready for the next entry of nurse request.

If a patient is transferred to another clinical area, and if the computers in the hospital are linked via a networking system, then the information about the patient, coded according to the patient's hospital number, can be accessed by the admitting ward or clinical area using the appropriate password.

Likewise, patients who wish to be involved in the production of their own care plans can do this using the FIP system, because they too can choose information, problems, outcomes and interventions from the library in the same way as the nurse. The information simply has to be read from the screen, and if it is not quite right it can be edited. Because this is a more visual activity than normal collaborative care planning activity, and also because the FIP system is colour-coded – so that, for instance, whenever the package is dealing with problems the information is highlighted in red, and each of the other stages have different colours – it becomes easier for the patient to see for himself what is going on. It also stimulates discussion about the use of the computer. One other benefit from this system, which should be present in any effective care planning system, is the ability to see all the stages on the computer screen at any one time so that both patient and nurse can see how the care plan is building up. Again, these should be colour-coded, as they are with the FIP system.

The FIP system can also be used to communicate with FIP's other computer packages. These include a community-based one, which is useful for patients being discharged to the community psychiatric nurse. However, the care planning system itself is also appropriate for the CPN, who might wish to maintain continuity and use the format on which the patient's care has already been formulated. Of course, when the patient has been discharged, the nursing team might wish to evaluate, retrospectively, the whole of the care course in an attempt to find out what was effective and what was not, for the benefit of future patients. The FIP Care Planning System allows the nurse to print out the whole of the care plans and related information on the patient or, if necessary, specific parts of it. The data itself can be interrogated so that nurses can find out how much of a particular style, intervention or problem was present at any one time.

A fast developing area in CACP is the use of programmes on a mobile basis. A big criticism of CACP has always been that it can only be carried out in the ward office or nursing station. However, with the advent of 'portables' – powerful computers that can be carried around – the nurse is now able to take the computer to the patient rather than vice–versa, and to work on the care programme wherever is most convenient. This has particular significance for the community nurse who can take the portable around with her all day and then down load the information into the main computer when she returns to the office. Of course, the software has to enable this function to be carried out, and the FIP system does this without any difficulty, though the needs and costs of portable systems have to be carefully worked out.

As can be seen, there are certain key factors to be considered in the selection of an effective CACP system, and the FIP Care Planning System has been used as an example of what can be achieved with a little thought and application. Computers may never actually replace the nurse's manual production of a care plan but they should certainly be seen as a method of combining the advantages of human flexibility and technological specificity to produce an approach which has many attributes, not least of which are speed of use and access to large libraries of relevant information. Certainly, the continuity offered by such a system would be difficult to match using traditional manual activities.

PATIENT INVOLVEMENT

It may often be difficult actually to include the patient in this planning phase, but in cases where it is possible it is of great therapeutic value if he can be encouraged to contribute his own ideas. Allowing the patient to explore the strategies concerning the resolution of his difficulties can only act as a reinforcer for his eventual successful actions. Remember, the nurse is not trying to make the patient dependent upon her, but independent of her. He must be fully aware of what is to happen and how best to use activities for his own sake. Highly technical terminology should be avoided at all costs as it only confuses the patient and creates an aura of mystery around his own care. He must be aware of the steps by which he progresses so that he can use them as building blocks for the future. They may well involve considerable hard work on the patient's part so he must be able to see the point of it all. Before initiating the care plan, it is best to approach the patient and discuss it with him, seeking his approval. In this way, he becomes a participant in the process and not just the object of it.

CASE STUDY: JULIE DAWSON

The type of nursing intervention used in the case study may not necessarily be that which the reader would use. Different approaches will reflect experience, type of training and the methods or strategies that the individual nurse has been exposed to. Here, the approach, the method of documentating and the attention to detail will be of greater value than the actual intervention itself. The suggested reader exercise will enable readers to express their own personal intervention in the way they think best, but also following the pattern as laid down in the examples. It will be noted that the care is separated into its various components and each sub-heading given a separate letter code. In this way, as with the problem and objective coding, the care can be referred to easily at a later date by its coding, i.e. (3b)

or (2a) etc. It will also be noted that no element of the care given by the nurse is regarded as too elementary or unimportant to document. Carrying half the care around in her head is not the way for the nurse to promote continuity and provide total care.

Two separate care plans are given for Julie Dawson (Figs 6.1 and 6.2). Only the right sides of the care plans are illustrated, so it will be necessary to refer back to Chapter 5 for diagnoses/objective data. In Chapter 8 we will discuss the evaluation procedure and combine the two plans at that point.

READER EXERCISE

Complete the following case plan for Susan (Fig. 6.3). Refer to Chapters 3–5 for background to the case study.

SUMMARY

The nursing process as a method of delivering nursing care is a scientific approach but within the care planning component the nurse is offered the opportunity to express herself in a creative fashion. In this way she is able to both humanise nursing interventions and combine this with her knowledge of the mechanics of human behaviour to enhance her future effectiveness. The nurse must, however, remain within the structure of the system. This involves following a very definite pattern of action whereby the nurse isolates what it is she hopes to achieve before stating the methods and means by which she hopes to achieve it. If this pattern is not followed, the care delivered may well be damaging to the patient's welfare. Equally, if the care is not documented for all nursing personnel to refer to, patient contact may well become fragmented and inconsistent. This lack of continuity will not only hamper the patient's progress but may even exacerbate the symptoms he presents. One final word of caution for the discerning reader: the most successful methods of care within the psychiatric discipline are usually the simplest ones involving the minimum of staff. When planning care, always try to implement those approaches which are both easy to use and easy to understand.

Primary nurse: Karen Walters		Sheet number: 1	
Nursing interventions	Evaluations	Date	Nurse's initials
a) Establish sleep pattern and chart. b) Increase sleep areas by reducing stimuli at designated times. c) Encourage warm drink prior to sleep. d) Promote sleep routine.			
a) Assigned nurse to introduce herself to Julie at ½ hourly intervals. b) Ask one question about her feelings. c) Use empathy to explore the way she looks.			
a) Encourage exploration of ward by leaving her door open. b) Discuss ward excursion at least once every hour. c) Discourage early return to ward by diverting her – do not force her and provide active reinforcement when she does walk about. d) Discuss ward geography.			

Fig. 6.1 Julie Dawson's interim care plan (Care Plan 1).

Primary nurse: ..*Karen Walters*.......... Sheet number: ..*2*...............

Nursing interventions	Evaluations	Date	Nurse's initials
② a) Increase contact to all team members. b) Produce roster for nurse conversation. c) Ensure contact each time till contact acknowledged by Julie. d) Document discussed conversation content.			
③ a) Increase toilet time to 2 mins. b) Introduce to other patients. c) Offer a drink whilst on excursion. d) Offer congratulations if she stays out of room for long period of time.			
④ a) Discuss making list at beginning of shift b) State time to discuss list. c) Remind her of the list at regular times during the shift - ie ½ hourly at first. d) Try to get her to expand on why items appear on list.			
⑤ a) Encourage a basin wash before bath. b) If Julie requests a bath at any time - agree. c) Try to suggest bath at same time each day to establish a routine. Ask Julie which time would be best.			
⑥ a) Ensure that one of her excursions coincides with refreshment breaks. b) If possible leave her in the company of other patients and observe discreetly.			

Fig. 6.2 Julie Dawson's on-going care plan (Care Plan 2).

Primary nurse: ....   Sheet number: ....

Nursing interventions	Evaluation	Date	Nurse's initials

Fig. 6.3 Reader exercise: Susan's care plan (for completion).   © Longman Group UK Limited 1992

REFERENCES

FIP 1991 Newland House, 139 Hagley Road, Birmingham, England
Marriner A 1979 Planning. In: The nursing process: a scientific approach to nursing care. C.V. Mosby, St Louis
Meades S 1989 Integrative care planning in acute psychiatry. Journal of Advanced Nursing 14: 630–639
Pesut D J 1989 Aim versus blame: using an outcome specification model. Journal of Psychosocial Nursing and Mental Health Services 27(5): 26–30
Ward M F, Bishop R 1986 Learning to care in community psychiatric nursing. Hodder & Stoughton, Sevenoaks
Waterworth S, Luker K A 1990 Reluctant collaborators: do patients want to be involved in decisions concerning care? Journal of Advanced Nursing 15(8): 971–976

SUGGESTED READING

Iwasiw C L, Sleightholm-Cairns B 1990 Clinical conferences: the key to successful experiential learning. Nurse Education Today 10: 260–265
McHugh M 1986 Nursing process: musings on the method. Holistic Nursing Practice 1(1): 21–28
Reed R C 1989 Chaining nursing diagnosis: the use of etiological sequencing in the development of a care plan. Archives of Psychiatric Nursing 3(6): 344–350
Quinsland L K, van Ginkel A 1984 How to process experience. Journal of Experiential Education 7(2): 8–13

7

Implementation

INTRODUCTION

The nurse is ready at this point to implement the planned care she has outlined for her patient. It is an exciting prospect because she is putting her skills to the test. If she and her patient are to be successful in achieving their objectives, then the care plan must be adhered to as closely as possible. It would be unwise to say that they must stick to it rigidly, because this is not always possible. It is unrealistic to suppose that every aspect of a care plan can be implemented with every patient at all times. The unpredictable nature of nursing psychiatric patients does not allow for everything to run smoothly, and if situations arise beyond the nurse's control in the form of crises, admissions or staff shortages, she must be prepared to adapt to them. Eventually, the care plan will have to be evaluated, and the amount of time spent with the patient in relation to the resources available within the clinical area will constitute a major part of that evaluation. The nurse must work hard to establish plans which offer her room for manoeuvre should extraneous interferences warrant it.

Of course, when a situation arises which prevents the nurse from carrying out her intervention, she must have at her disposal a method of reporting this information and assessing the problems she has encountered. Effective management of time cannot be evaluated unless it has been documented. It is also necessary to have data related to the patient's response to care, the people who have been involved in its administration, when and how it was carried out and a record of its actual delivery. For this reason, care plans must be accompanied by patient progress notes.

PROGRESS NOTES

These notes are not the diary of events usually associated with nursing documentation, but a statement of the relevant information surrounding the delivery of a patient's care (Bower 1982, Jones 1984). They are initiated as soon as the patient is admitted and give a detailed account of his stay whilst in the clinical area. It is important that they are written in such a way as to plot changes that take place within the therapeutic sequence. Repetitive statements, such as 'slept well', 'slept well', 'slept well', are of no value. Entries must have significance and be pertinent and objective. Progress notes are designed to complement the care plan, not act as an alternative to it. Their other major function is to illustrate the daily activities of the patient in relation to his care environment. The therapy provided by the nurse on her plan forms only part of the total picture, and it is in the progress notes that all the relevant data concerning the patient is recorded (Pothier 1988). Ideally they should be stored with the care plans so that the link between (1) what is to be done, and (2) what has happened is easily monitored.

WHO WRITES IN THE PROGRESS NOTES?

Two major factors must be considered – professionalism and accountability.

Professionalism

If the progress notes are to follow an expected pattern and make a real contribution to the patient's documentation, they should only be written by, or under the supervision of, a trained member of staff. All too often, notes are written by untrained staff whose unscientific approach falls far short of the standards required of the professional nurse. Examples of this are:

- notes written simply because nothing has been documented in the patient's progress notes for several days
- repetitive notes written on the principle that, 'if it was the case yesterday, it must be the case today'
- trivia
- inconsequential, over-inclusive discussions
- subjective opinions
- criticisms
- hearsay or uncorroborated information.

Accountability

It is the responsibility of the senior nurse on each shift to monitor what is written in the progress notes, though it is certainly not necessary for her actually to write them. Ultimately, what is written will reflect the influence of that senior nurse and help to establish a pattern that can be used as both a teaching medium for nursing students and a structured comparison for qualified junior staff. The foundation for accurate and informative progress notes is as scientifically based as that of the nursing process itself, and untrained support staff cannot be expected to fulfil this nursing obligation without supervision. As such supervision cannot always be offered, it is necessary for trained staff, and especially those working as key workers with particular patients, to vet information before it is written down and to document it themselves because they must take responsibility for it. It is impossible for the ward sister or charge nurse to exercise any degree of control or continuity if the staff completing the notes are not consciously influenced by the nursing philosophy that governs their actions (Lambertson 1988).

RECORDING INFORMATION

Regardless of whether patient information and progress are documented by trained staff or learners, they need to identify clearly what it is they intend to report, and how they are going to report it. In psychiatry, the majority of nursing activities centre around non-physical methods of delivering care, so it follows that the patient's progress notes will contain a considerable amount of behavioural observations related to interpersonal actions. The nursing process itself is a method of establishing a therapeutic link between the patient and the nurse, and much of what happens during that contact is of far greater value than the procedure through which it is taking place. This personal element is difficult both to record and to evaluate in terms of its effect on the patient. However, the nurse must have this information at her disposal if she is to evaluate her care correctly and plan future intervention in accordance with it. She needs a system of reporting that will fulfil several major requirements:

- It must be adaptable to both the independent and dependent actions she must make.
- It must show how the nursing process activities relate to the regular or standard care that is provided.
- It must provide a readily accessible source of information to all members of the multidisciplinary team who wish to refer to it.
- It must follow a pattern.
- It must be easy to use.
- It must show the relation between the care delivered and the patient's response to it.
- It must only document change.
- It must be objective.
- It should act as a teaching tool whereby all who refer to it learn something about the patient, his situation, his care or his progress (or deterioration).

The only system which is capable of accommodating all these requirements was developed under the title of problem-oriented recording (POR), as outlined by Weed (1968) and later adapted to psychiatry by Grant & Maletzky (1972). Like the nursing process, POR is a system by which patient information is collected, assessed, acted upon and recorded, but our main concern here is with its system of recording. The format described by Weed (1971) is that of SOAP notes.

SOAP NOTES

SOAP is an abbreviation for the elements contained within each of the entries in the POR system. These are:

- *Subjective*: what the patient says, or what someone else says relating to the patient.
- *Objective*: the direct observation of the situation made by the nurse, i.e. what she sees.
- *Assessment*: a conclusion drawn from the information the nurse has gained.
- *Plan*: what the nurse intends to do, if anything.

SOAP notes are written each time a change takes place in any one of these four areas, and they are particularly suitable in psychiatric nursing for the recording of psychosocial information. Weed maintained that all grades of staff, both medical and nursing, should use the format. Cormack (1980) recommended that SOAP notes should be used instead of a care plan. Cormack includes an 'expected outcome' section at the end of his record, thus converting the whole system into a nursing process, except that it is anticlockwise. However, when documentated it is not easy to pick up what needs to be done, when, where and in what way. As an action document the SOAP format is therefore open to abuse, but as a complementary one for the nursing process it is ideal.

SOAP notes examples

The general approach to the use of the system can best be understood by looking at some examples and, in particular, at the way the information is expressed.

Example one

A simple example might look like this:

Subjective: Jane refused mid-day medication and said that she did not want it.
Objective: Became alarmed and distressed.
Assessment: Doesn't usually refuse medication, but I have only recently met Jane and she doesn't know me well.

Plan: I will spend some time with her so that she feels more confident in my company, and ask her to take her medication later.

The change evident, here, is that Jane usually takes her medication but today she has refused. The nurse decides from her behaviour that it has something to do with her approach with the medication and she elects to rectify the situation by becoming better acquainted with Jane and trying her with the medication later.

Her plan could have followed several other paths depending on her assessment. She could have:

- asked another member of staff to offer Jane her medication
- concluded that Jane's behaviour was due to an increase in her psychiatric symptomatology and spent more time discussing that problem with her
- decided she had no idea why Jane refused and planned to find out why.

Example two

In some situations the plan itself may simply follow what one might expect in the circumstances.

Subjective: Alan appeared on the ward at 2300 hours stating he was fed up with being in hospital.
Objective: Could hardly stand up unsupported; speech slurred and smelling of alcohol.
Assessment: Appeared heavily intoxicated. Has done this before, twice in the last week and usually after he has been visited by his wife. This is probably a reaction to the stress he feels following these visits.
Plan: 1.   Will encourage him to go to bed as soon as possible.
       2.   Will monitor his level of consciousness at 30-minute intervals during the night.
       3.   Will ask day staff to confront him with his method of dealing with this situation.

Example three

In some instances the nurse may not necessarily know what plan of action to take, and this will be reflected in her record.

Subjective: Mrs Holbrooke says that someone keeps going into her room and she doesn't see the need for it.
Objective: Lies in bed and refuses to speak to anyone.
Assessment: Has still not managed to come to terms with her active delusional system and doesn't accept her hospital environment for what it is. Is probably frightened by her experiences.
Plan: Continue with care plan activities. Problem 2.

It will be seen from all of these examples that little time has elapsed between the situation occurring and it being documented. It may not always be possible for the nurse to report what she has seen immediately after it has happened, but she must make great efforts to complete a written record of her actions in relation to her patient and the patient's response in relation to her.

Points to remember whilst making SOAP patient progress notes are:

- Avoid the use of too many technical terms; keep it as straightforward as possible.
- Date and sign each entry that is made, possibly giving the time also.
- Each element of the record should be completed even if it only emphasises the need for further investigation.
- The nurse must attempt to do something in each situation and with each entry. This may not always be appropriate but in the majority of cases some nursing intervention will be warranted.
- The reason or rationale for intervention should be clearly expressed, usually in the assessment element.
- Write it down as soon as possible.

Example four

SOAP notes are a method of documenting a patient's progress but in the first three examples only single entries were given. The following is a progress record as it might appear in the nursing notes. The value of this example is in the documentation process it follows rather than in the actions taken, which not everyone may agree with.

19/11/91 S: David says that all of us are against him and want to make him look silly.

O: Was shouting and screaming in the day area. Swearing at the female patients.

A: Refuses to express his feelings in a more acceptable fashion.

P: 1. Refer to Care Plan Problem 3
2. Talk to him about his feelings concerning his behaviour on the ward.

C/N Jones.

19/11/91: S: David says he is very angry with the ward staff.

17.15 h O: Struck Nurse Johnson on the face at tea-time after she had asked him to help clear the dining tables.

A: Seems to feel more threatened by female staff than by male staff.

P: 1. Get male staff to speak to him this evening.
2. Assign male staff to his care plan for the remainder of the day.

C/N Jones.

20/11/91 S: David refuses to take part in the group activities because he says they are silly.

O: Ran off the ward at 11.00 hours shouting and gesticulating. Returned 10 minutes later and refused to speak to anyone.

A: Still finds it difficult to respond in an acceptable fashion to his own feelings, in particular with potentially threatening situations.

P: 1. Continue with Care Plan Activity Problem 3.
2. Encourage to attend this afternoon's group meeting.

S/N Bird.

20/11/91 S: Enjoyed ward group meeting.

O: Participated throughout the meeting and did not become too agitated when confronted by his own behaviour.

A: Is prepared to think about his behaviour only if he sees it as being masculine to do so. Feels he has gained a small victory this afternoon.

P: 1. To confront him with the effects of his behaviour using drama therapy methods whenever he becomes hostile.
2. Remain sympathetic towards him.
3. This work initially to be carried out by male staff.
4. Continue with Care Plan Activity Problem 3 which is up for review tomorrow.

SR Mason.

Problem 3 on the care plan in this case refers to problems of communication, David's objective being that at the end of one week he is able to discuss any anti-social behaviour he exhibits without shouting at the nurse. The progress notes have confirmed his behaviour, demonstrated how it manifests itself and also highlighted a possible precipitating cause – that of his relationship towards females, especially those recognized as being in authority. It is easy to see how the link between the care and the SOAP notes is maintained. Likewise, it is easy to see that during the initial stages of the nursing process, i.e. during observation and assessment, the careful compilation of complementary progress notes is a vital tool for gaining a better understanding of the patient's situation, his problems and his responses to them.

WHEN TO WRITE THE PROGRESS NOTES

It is impossible to place a time limit on the entries each patient requires. For some it may be every three or four days, for others a matter of minutes only. As each clinical situation is different so too will be the appropriate recording time. The one most important aspect about these records, however, is that they are written because there is a need to do so, not because it is just another task that the nursing staff have to perform. There is no place for task-oriented progress notes. Senior staff who allocate one nurse to complete all the records for a whole shift, or who say to a nurse during the latter stages of a shift 'go do the notes' are really wasting a lot of people's time. Likewise, assigned staff who feel obligated to write in the progress notes at the end of each period of duty are also denying their patients the right to active and efficient documentation, and their multi-disciplinary team members their need for quality information (Walker & Selmanoff 1964). An ideal opportunity to help their patients is being thrown away if they do not accurately plot those incidents which have meaning and significance. If everything is logged and recorded the important element becomes lost in a page of repetitive and routine subjectivity and professional gossip. It will never be read; it will never be acted upon; thus it is wasted. There are of course, several reasons why nurses do not document anything in the patient's progress notes:

- they have nothing to say about them
- nothing unusual has happened – no change or progress
- they do not know who the patient is
- they have avoided the patient for a variety of reasons
- the patient has avoided them, also for a variety of reasons.

All these points should be considered when it is noted that an entry has not been made in the notes for a reasonable period of time. It is fair to assume that patients who demand care will have more entries than those who do not. By definition, this means that one can expect more entries in an acute admission area than in a medium or long-stay area; with the elderly mentally ill, the situation may oscillate from one extreme to the other. Ultimately, it is up to each senior nurse to decide whether or not adequate documentary evidence is available regarding their individual patients, and if not they must find out why.

ADMINISTRATION OF CARE

The actual delivery of care is not an appropriate subject for this book, but its administration is. Having spent considerable time gathering a database, formulating a patient profile, assessing the problems and finally planning the care, it would be foolish to assume that the care plans simply went into the patient's folder and were acted upon as if by magic. Care has to be administered in the same way as it is planned – systematically and scientifically. The management of the care plan is the responsibility of the senior nurse on the ward. Only she is aware of the resources and facilities that exist in her area at any one time, and therefore only she can correctly assess how best to allocate nursing activities. There are several methods that may be used; all have their particular attributes and may be appropriate to only a certain set of circumstances.

Method one: shift allocation

Under this method the senior nurse reallocates the care plans to her staff every day on a supply and demand basis, i.e. if there are three staff and 15 care plans, they each get five to deal with, but not necessarily the same five as they had the previous shift.

Good points

- Each member of staff becomes familiar with all the patients after only a few days.
- Each patient has a variety of staff fulfilling his nursing requirements.
- The senior nurse is not tied down to rigid allocation systems.

Bad points

- Patients do not get the opportunity to establish a strong working relationship with individual nurses.
- Nurses become confused about what they are supposed to be achieving with each patient.
- Patients may feel that they are pawns in a professional game and consider themselves to be simply observers of ward routine.

Method two: weekly allocation

Here, the care plans are allocated on a weekly basis. Nurses receive a set of care plans for which they are responsible for a seven-day period irrespective of their shift commitments.

Good points

- A degree of stability is introduced into the delivery of care because each patient spends a reasonable amount of time with his respective nurse and a relationship is allowed to develop.
- Both patients and staff benefit from the relationship, because of the greater understanding of each other.
- Progress notes are of a higher quality because the allocated nurse has a better assessment base from which to work.

Bad points

- Because it is a rigid allocation system, serious faults arise if the allocated nurse becomes ill or is absent for any reason.
- When the nurse is off duty the plans have to be re-allocated, and the nurse to whom this happens then has an extra case load to deal with.
- If senior staff act as stand-ins for absent staff, the delivery of care may be hampered by their other managerial duties.
- The patient may not like the nurse to whom he is allocated.

Method three: rota admission allocation

On admission each patient is allocated to a nurse. That nurse becomes responsible for the whole of the care process including observation, assessment and care planning. No attempt is made to match nurse to patient, just a strict rota which depends solely on who is present when the patient arrives.

Good points

- The nurse allocated to the patient has an excellent opportunity to build a worthwhile relationship.
- Through this relationship she gains a far greater understanding of the patient's problems, needs and capabilities and is, therefore, more motivated to create enlightened care plans.
- The patient feels attached to a particular nurse whom he can identify at any time.
- Senior staff do not have to worry about sorting out allocations because the system is rigidly adhered to.

Bad points

- The same problems exist for time-off cover as for the previous two methods.
- Some staff feel it is an unfair allocation method as one nurse might develop larger case loads than others simply because of their presence during admissions.
- If the rota system works in the nurse's absence, i.e. on a strict rotational basis irrespective of shifts, it may be as long as two or three days before the patient actually meets the nurse to whom he is allocated.
- The patient may easily become too dependent on the one nurse.

Method four: team allocation

Ward staff are split into teams, a representative of which is present on each shift. Each shift receives equal allocation on a rotation system and the patient receives the care from whichever representative is present on the shift.

Good points

- Each patient always has a nurse familiar with his particular care plan and background on each shift.
- No break in continuity through time-off, though sickness may still present a problem.
- Allocation method is easy for senior staff, who might not actually be involved with any of the teams.
- The patient has a team to relate to rather than one nurse and, therefore, has less chance of becoming too dependent on one individual.
- All staff dealing with the patient are familiar with the pre-planning details of the patient's care.

Bad points

- On areas where there are small staffing levels, the team system cannot work because there simply are not enough people to put into teams that will cover each shift.
- Poor inter-shift communication may seriously hamper the transfer of relevant details from one representative to another.

Method five: primary nursing

This system is extensively used in the USA. It is similar to team nursing except that each team may consist of as little as two people, one of whom is trained and acts as the primary nurse, and the other or others who are junior or untrained and act as associate nurses. The primary nurse is responsible for the administration, the planning and the evaluation of the care plans, and aiding in the care delivery process. The associate nurse carries out the activities of the care plan, reporting information to the leader. Multidisciplinary staff wishing for information regarding the patient receive it from the primary nurse, who is responsible for her workload throughout the patient's period of hospitalisation. Senior ward personnel act as advisors and liaison offi-

cers, being ultimately responsible for all primary nursing teams and the care loads (Mutchner 1986).

Individual nurses, either primary or associate, may act as key workers for patients within their care group. They provide specific skills or therapy for these selected patients, or have developed good relationships with them that have enabled a therapeutic link to develop to positive effect for the patients. Key workers should not work cross-group, but should only work with patients from their own care group.

Good points

- Introduces junior staff to management activities and maintains their high level of involvement in work processes.
- Reduces the work load on sisters and charge nurses.
- Team leaders are more accessible to the individual patients.
- Continuity of care is maintained.
- Senior learners and junior qualified staff receive executive powers of action at an earlier stage in their professional development and therefore become more skilled in nursing techniques.
- Sisters and charge nurses are released for more supervisory activities.

Bad points

- Patient contact is reduced for sisters and charge nurses.
- Reasonable staffing levels are required to make the system work effectively, though not as many as are required for simple team allocation.
- Off-duty system becomes very rigid to ensure one member of the nursing team is on duty at all times.
- Head nurses may still have to stand in for sickness breaks.
- Team members must be prepared to cover for each other.
- If the team members do not get on well, patient care may suffer because of the conflict.

- Patients may feel they are getting second class care because the sister or charge nurse does not seem to be directly in control of their programme.

Although psychiatric nursing traditionally suffers from low staffing levels, in particular with trained staff, primary nursing is probably the best method of care plan allocation, and care delivery. It offers greater involvement in many different areas for both staff and patients, and facilitates a greater interplay between scientific and creative elements of care. Just as importantly, it allows staff to carry out their designated roles, much as their job descriptions intended. It may not be possible to institute primary nursing as soon as the nursing process is implemented; senior staff may have to progress through other methods of allocation as the situation dictates. However, it should be the eventual aim of the senior ward manager to be able to deliver care using this method of administration.

PATIENT INVOLVEMENT

While care plan administration may be the responsibility of the nurses on the ward, the implementation of that care is very much a shared responsibility – shared between the patient and the nurse. In an ideal situation, it is shared three ways: between the patient, his relatives and the nurse. In psychiatry, particularly, it is important that the patient's relatives become involved in the planning and implementation of care as in many situations they may be one of the causes of the patient's behaviour. It is imperative that they are involved so that:

- they acquire a better understanding of the patient's problems and his particular method of dealing with them
- the patient sees a caring commitment from those people in his environment who provide stability and security for him, and yet with whom he may well have difficulty in relating.

If the patient grows through the help of his relatives as well as that of the professional staff

he has a much better chance of recovery and, in a reciprocal fashion, his relatives too will have a better understanding of how to help him solve his problems in the future without recourse to hospital admission.

The nurse can ensure that the patient is involved in his care by:

- keeping him informed of his progress
- reminding him of his objectives
- asking him about how he feels towards the care he is receiving
- asking his advice about the effects of his care
- pointing out recognised areas of difficulty and counselling him in ways of finding alternative approaches
- discussing failures in depth to establish what went wrong and providing support and encouragement for future schemes
- ensuring that he is aware of the activity he is supposed to be involved in
- asking him to be critical of his behaviour
- helping him to be constructive in his approach to the appraisal of his own achievements
- asking him what changes might be necessary and allowing him to be present at evaluation sessions where possible and appropriate.

This last item will be dealt with in the next chapter, but it is important to note that the patient's inclusion in all aspects of managing his care, and planning the necessary intervention, is an essential component in his successful recovery. The main feature of the patient's involvement is the communication that takes place between him and his nurses, be they team leaders, daily allocated staff, evaluation committees or head nurses. That communication must at all times be a two-way process maintained to a very high degree.

SUMMARY

This chapter has not been about the care that is delivered to the patient but about the support methods that may be employed to ensure that the machinery by which it is presented is effective and efficient. The complementary activity of producing progress notes and the advocation of the

SOAP note format for its objectivity and accuracy were discussed. Meaningful patient progress notes are essential if careful monitoring of the effect of care delivery is to be carried out and both dependent and independent nursing functions are to be documentated in a way which highlights their interdependence. The different methods of allocating care plans were discussed and, once again, a particular approach suitable to the psychiatric discipline that might be the eventual aim of senior ward staff – that of primary nursing – was discussed. Finally, the involvement of the patient and his relatives in the delivery of his own care was considered. It may have been more appro-

priate to place that section at the beginning of the chapter because, in truth, no matter how you view psychiatric nursing, if the patient is not involved in his own care and the solving of his own problems, the nurse is merely indulging in self-gratification and the satisfaction of her own needs as a nurse. Nursing care can only be effective if it is offered and received by mutual agreement, and that can only be achieved if it is understood and accepted by the patient. Therefore, the communication component contained within this section of the nursing process remains of paramount importance to the nurse if she is to create a suitable environment for adaptability or recovery.

REFERENCES

Bower F L 1982 The process of planning nursing care. Nursing practice models, 3rd edn. C V Mosby, St Louis
Cormack D 1980 The nursing process. An application of the SOAP model. Nursing Times 76: 12 Occasional Paper
Grant R, Maletzky B 1972 Application of the Weed system to psychiatric records. Psychiatry in Medicine 3: 123
Jones L M 1984 Process recording for communication with psychiatric patients: techniques for improving skills of communication. In: Faulkner A (ed) Communication – recent advances in nursing series. Churchill Livingstone, Edinburgh
Lambertson E C 1988 Forces influencing the delivery of nursing services. In: Krebbs M J, Larson K (eds) Applied

psychiatric – mental health standards in clinical practice. John Wiley & Son, New York, Ch. 13
Mutchner L L 1986 How well are we practising primary nursing? Journal of Nursing Administration 16(9): 8–13
Pothier P C 1988 Let others know what you are doing. Archives of Psychiatric Nursing 3: 125
Walker V H, Selmanoff E D 1964 A study of the nature and use of nursing notes. Nursing Research, 8 August: 113–121
Weed L L 1968 Medical records that guide and teach. New England Journal of Medicine 278(11): 593–599, 652–657
Weed L L 1971 Preparing and maintaining the problem-orientated record: the PROMIS method. The Press of Case Western Reserve University, Virginia

SUGGESTED READING

Allen H 1987 Voices of concern: a study of verbal communication about patients in a psychiatric day unit. Journal of Advanced Nursing 6: 355–362
Chapman G E 1988 Reporting therapeutic discourse in a therapeutic community. Journal of Advanced Nursing 13(2): 255–264

Fow-Unger E, Wewell G, Guilbault K 1989 Documentation: communicating professionalism. Nurse Management 20(1): 65–70
Woolley F R, Warnick M W, Kane R L, Dyer E D 1974 Problem orientated nursing. Springer, New York

8

Evaluation

INTRODUCTION

The nursing process is a cyclical approach to nursing intervention. True, it has a beginning, that of the initial observation period, but as it progresses through its various sections it returns to the assessment element once again. Here, decisions are made about the care given, the patient's responses to it and the suitability of alternatives. It is a reassessment of the patient's situation, only now the nurse has far more relevant information at her disposal and can gain a greater insight into the patient's potential for recovery. This reassessment phase is known as 'evaluation'. Evaluation may involve changing elements of the patient's care plan or carrying on as originally planned. It therefore makes the process a dynamic one in that it is never ending. Evaluation of nursing care is vital because it ensures that the nurse continues to monitor patient progress in relation to the care given, adapting problems, objectives and interventions in accordance with her observations. Failure to evaluate will ultimately produce unsatisfactory, uncontrolled and uncoordinated nursing intervention, possibly inappropriate to the changing needs of the patient. Evaluation times are pre-set by the period allowed for each short-term objective, and the information for executive decisions about the care plan is gained from the continuous observation inherent in psychiatric nursing. The evaluation statements – whether about the success of achieving an objective, the difficulties encountered in failing to do so, or the need for care plan modification – must be recorded; in the case of the care plan used in this book it will be on the plan itself.

Nursing care itself is measured in terms of its quality; it is not an analysis of the tasks involved. Thus, evaluation also becomes a method of quality control (Vogel 1988). To achieve this, however, evaluative assessment must go far beyond merely gauging the effectiveness of the patient's care plans. This chapter is therefore an indispensible part of the book.

Evaluation involves three elements:

1. The nursing intervention given by the nurse responsible for planning and implementing care. This is sometimes called the concurrent nursing audit.
2. Patient progress in relation to his short-term and long-term objectives. This will nearly always involve some form of care plan modification.
3. The total intervention offered to a patient by the nursing staff during his period of hospitalisation or in each nursing department. This may involve two separate audits, for instance where community nurses are involved in the after-care of the patient. Zimmer (1976) called this the retrospective nursing audit.

CONCURRENT NURSING AUDIT

There are several ways in which a continuous evaluation of the nurse's effectiveness may be achieved. Some involve the professional skills of senior nursing personnel, both in formal and informal situations. Others simply require the nurse to keep a check on her own activity. The following are a sample of the approaches that might be incorporated into the ward routines:

- self-analysis and evaluation
- informal discussions with senior nursing staff, either sisters or charge nurses
- ward staff meetings
- peer discussions
- team discussion (in the case of team/primary nursing approaches)

- monitoring by teaching staff
- discussion by nurse audit committees.

SELF-EVALUATION

It is primarily the responsibility of the nurse who had planned the care to evaluate it. However, this is only part of the story for it is very difficult for a person who is deeply committed and involved in her work to objectively assess her own performance. Self-analysis of her approach to her delivery of care is important to the nurse for several reasons.

- It provides insight into her own effectiveness. The nurse's opinion of herself often has a far greater influence on her future activities than a hundred suggestions from sisters, charge nurses and clinical teachers.
- It reminds her that she is an integral part of the patient's treatment while he finds difficulty in dealing with his own life situation. Without her, he may never return to personal competency.
- If she is truly critical of her actions, it ensures that the quality of her responses to the patient are maintained at a high level.
- For the psychiatric nurse it is vital that she is able to function well both in a team and in an independent role, and the confidence necessary for this responsible approach can be achieved through a systematic appraisal of her own actions.

For the nurse to ask herself 'was that done correctly?' is a good place to start the evaluative process but it is hardly enough. What she needs are criteria for self-evaluation outlined in a series of questions she can ask herself at regular chosen intervals (McFarlane 1982). The following is one approach to the check list. Have I:

- Carried out the care required by the patient's care plan?
- Observed the effects of the care given?
- Communicated all necessary information to the patient regarding his care?
- Recorded all relevant information during the intervention period?
- Kept other staff informed of care effects?

- Asked the patient about his feelings towards the care he is receiving?
- Taken steps to modify the care given where it is inappropriate?
- Identified the changing need pattern of the patient and modified the care plan accordingly?
- Developed a creative approach with the planned framework?
- Maintained a good working relationship with the patient, retaining my professionalism while meeting his nursing requirements?
- Been effective in my approach to the care I gave?

And finally,

- Could I have done better?

With the exception of the last one the answer to all the questions in the check list should at all times be 'yes'; if it is not, the situation should be analysed to see what can be done to produce a positive response.

INFORMAL DISCUSSIONS

In the majority of psychiatric establishments, the relationship between all grades of staff, though professional, is very much an informal one. This encourages interaction between all those concerned with patient care, and creates a good work atmosphere within the clinical area. It is inevitable that out of this system a method of informal evaluation by senior staff should grow. Basically, it is the responsibility of senior trained staff to monitor the activity of those people working within their team, and one of the areas that can act as a useful guide to their progress is that of evaluating their actions in relation to the nursing process.

The same criteria can be used as for self-evaluation except that it is the sister or charge nurse who asks the questions, and then compares the answers given by the nurse involved with their own knowledge and expertise concerning the situation prevailing within the ward. Advice on alternative strategies, new ideas or simple congratulations offered on a one-to-one basis without the constraints of a formal investigation can reap remarkable benefits. The nurse feels that her work has importance if others are prepared to sit down and discuss it objectively. The senior nurse is able to establish the strengths and weaknesses of her staff, and has the opportunity to mould and shape them so that they function as autonomous practitioners within a team framework. The benefits for the patient of such inter-staff communication should be easily apparent.

Randomly chosen quiet moments in the ward routine should be selected to review the care plans and their implications for the patient. These should not be confused with the more formal discussions that take place during the regular evaluations and modifications of the plans. Involvement is the key to good ward management, and learning situations will be greatly enhanced if it is seen that there is genuine interest and concern. Each member of the staff should be seen to have the same opportunities for an informal discussion, although if this is difficult with particular members of the team, other forms of evaluating their effectiveness may be necessary. Although it is the duty of senior staff to seek out their staff to offer their advice and help, this does not preclude those staff from seeking out the evaluation of their work if they are in need of help. It must be every nurse's responsibility to try to improve their intervention performance, as the patient can only benefit from this form of professional commitment.

WARD MEETINGS

Meetings at regular intervals are essential to the smooth running of a ward because they improve communication between the individual team members. Much can be discussed during these meetings and invariably they are kept on a relatively informal footing. A current evaluation of the effectiveness of the care that the team is providing should always be included in the discussion. Failure to identify problem areas at an early stage in their development may lead to almost insurmountable difficulties at a later date, often with dire consequences for the patients involved. The self-evaluation criteria discussed above can be used here too, but other elements must be included because questions need to be asked concerning the sociological impact of the team as a whole and not just of its individual members. For example:

● Does our intervention interfere with the activities of other departments or agencies involved on the ward?

● Are we creating a therapeutic atmosphere within the clinical area?

● Are we aware of what is expected of us in relation to care plan activities?

● How do we fit into the overall treatment programme outlined for individual patients?

● Do we understand what is happening to patients for whom we are not directly responsible on the ward?

● Are there other facilities or resources we could acquire that would improve our basic efficiency and effectiveness?

● Are we aware of new ideas and techniques that could be incorporated into our interventions with our patients?

● Are we managing our time as best as we possibly can?

As these meetings are often attended by nursing officers, patient care managers and representatives from other disciplines it is easy to see why these questions should be asked at this time. It may be possible to obtain instant feedback although future planning or research may be required. In any case, areas of need are brought out into the open and initial approaches towards tackling them can be brought into play. It must be remembered that the object of the exercise is to increase the quality of care provided, and as quality has no boundaries and cannot be measured in terms of its upper or outer limits it is essential that all avenues are explored. Areas that might be discussed could include problems involving disruptive patients, or communication with elderly mentally ill individuals or the effects of changing allocation patterns on the highly dependent patient. The effectiveness of the team providing the care can be measured to a degree in simple cause and effect terms: thus, if things

are going wrong on the ward it may be because of what the nurses are doing. A good cohesive team has a better chance than a disjointed unhappy one of producing a motivated patient community intent on recovery and all its rewards.

PEER DISCUSSIONS

Three basic areas involving peer discussion can be identified:

● trained staff interaction
● inter-learner teaching
● unit learner meetings.

Discussing her achievements, failures, problems and difficulties with her colleagues is nothing new to the nurse. Seeking advice is, after all, both a method of gaining support and a part of the self-evaluation process. For trained staff it may involve a few moments spent at handover comparing notes with their opposite number. For the learner, it may be slightly less informal, as senior learners could use the peer discussions as part of their teaching commitment to their juniors. In some cases, it might be possible to take this one step further and initiate a discussion group in which the learners from the unit could meet at regular intervals to examine their approach to their professional responsibilities. Such groups are growing in popularity within psychiatry, where the emphasis has always been on individual autonomy.

It must be stressed that peer evaluation is most effective when carried out in an informal setting involving staff of equal grades. The element of 'senior' and 'junior' is reduced considerably, thus facilitating a more personal appraisal of each individual's approach to her work.

Care assistants and auxiliaries should also be encouraged to discuss their activities with each other in the clinical situation. In most cases their only guidance comes from those who are more qualified than themselves, so that there is always an element of being told what to do. Peer discussion within this group may well give rise to a more honest evaluation of their work, thus enabling a greater degree of personal expression within the nursing team as a whole.

TEAM DISCUSSIONS

This kind of evaluation is more relevant to nurses using the team or primary nursing approach to care delivery. It could, however, be adapted for use by individual shifts or groups of nurses who regularly work together. The basic approach is very similar to that of the ward meetings except that what is evaluated is the effectiveness of the individual team in their own sphere of responsibility instead of the ward as a whole. The team may not necessarily consider the input of each member, but might evaluate areas such as:

- communication with other teams (shifts)
- team cohesiveness and morale
- team responsibilities
- case loads
- use of available resources and facilities
- multi-disciplinary communication
- problem areas
- reasons for both failure and success with a view to using that experience for future gain
- communication within the team itself
- small scale research into their own effectiveness.

Competition should be excluded from nursing at all costs, but a small element of team rivalry is not a bad thing if it involves taking pride in what is done. Regular meetings to discuss the team's effectiveness in all areas of care delivery should enhance both nurses' professionalism and team spirit. The patient can only benefit from the resultant increase in the nurse's motivation.

MONITORING BY NURSE EDUCATION STAFF

The nurse education department has an extremely important part to play in determining the quality of care that nurses provide. Their influence, however, can only be as great as their commitment within the clinical setting and to the learners working in it. It is not the intention to discuss the role of the teaching staff, as ultimately that will depend on their own philosophy and that of their schools and is, therefore, out of place in this book. (The nursing process and the education-

alist is, however, discussed in Chapter 14.) What is important here is how the teacher can aid the training nurse in her self-evaluation.

As is often the case in nurse education, and particularly in psychiatry, learners are allocated to a teacher or personal tutor throughout the whole of their training period. They therefore have the opportunity to develop a reasonable working relationship. If the teacher is to gain an insight into the activities of the learners and gauge their effectiveness as practising nurses she must work with them as much as possible in the clinical area. True, informal discussions within the confines and seclusion of the education department will aid the transmission of ideas and concepts; but it is an extremely imaginative learner who can perform independently of all guidance on the wards and still achieve a high degree of nursing competency as well as fulfilling her requisite team obligation. The following are some of the methods available to the teacher to enable her to gain the necessary evaluative information about the learner:

- Periods of supervisory nursing – not as an observer but as a participant.
- Ward reports – especially useful for the comments made by the senior staff, the identification of the learner's particular needs and for comparison at a later stage in the training.
- Inter-module appraisal – informal discussions with the learner and senior ward staff present. Ward reports are fine for a statement about the learner's overall performance, but if areas of difficulty can be identified during the interim periods ineffective or inappropriate nursing can be rectified before it has a chance to become accepted practice.
- Discussions with senior ward staff – between the teacher and the charge nurse or sister to establish whether there is any remedial activities that can be offered by the ward team.
- Discussion with a key worker.
- Discussions with team leaders.
- Discussions with primary nurses.
- Discussion with any supervising nurse working in the clinical area.
- Worksheets, projects and research related

to the activities that the learner is involved in. These are prepared to suit the student's particular requirements in the same way as the nursing process is designed to suit the individual patient.

● Completion of a work-related diary which must be produced to track a particular aspect of the student's clinical work.

● Monitoring the student's continuous assessment reviews.

Because the teacher has the scope to monitor learners over long periods of time she can help the learner to gain a more complete picture of her own effect on her patients, her colleagues and her professional activities. This evaluation procedure has the benefit of not demanding rapid results but, rather, allows the learner to develop her skills in the course of her own clinical experience. For this system to work efficiently, however, two elements are required.

1. The teacher must keep a record, either written or taped, of her evaluation of the learner's progress to use as a teaching aid throughout the training period.

2. The learner must keep some form of clinical diary connected with her own experience of the work situation, to use as an evaluation/comparison reference when working and when discussing her clinical approach with her teacher. This diary becomes both a teaching aid and a self-assessment tool when used with the evaluation criteria (Dietrich 1978).

NURSING AUDIT GROUPS I

It may be possible in some situations to establish a nursing audit committee responsible for monitoring the quality of the documentation of the nursing process. It must be stressed that such committees have no executive powers but only offer advice and guidance. Such a committee can be constituted from:

● unit nurse managers
● nurse teachers
● senior ward staff.

Preferably, each unit or group of wards has its own committee. Its role would be to:

● Examine a random sample of progress notes and give advice on their content and presentation.
● Examine nursing profiles and interview records to see if appropriate information has been recorded.
● Check care plans for evaluation dates, terminology and objective statements.
● Give advice on the care provided.
● Compare the documentation from different wards of the same classification, i.e. acute, continuing care etc., to see if improvements can be made or lessons learnt from similar difficulties experienced on those wards.
● Recommend improvements in documenting information.
● Conduct small scale research and examine new methods of nursing process activities (Lauri 1982).
● Identify problem areas and offer assistance in their solutions.

The idea of committees examining nurses' work is perhaps a little threatening in principle, but if the system is tackled realistically and with the involvement of as many staff as possible it is an excellent method of quality control. Everyone is capable of making errors and very often it is difficult to see where one is going wrong. Technical advice from colleagues can often throw light on difficult cases. Nurses, like all other health care professionals, must be confident enough in their own activities to allow scrutiny of their work so that they can learn from their own mistakes.

EVALUATION OF CARE PLANS

This element of the evaluation procedure is connected as much with the nursing objectives as with those of the patient. The nurse needs to establish that the care plan is being prepared in the most effective way, and this includes having evaluation information on the actual care plan so that it can be directly related to the care activity. What is important here is not the evaluation of the care plan in relation to patient activity but in relation to nursing activity. This is carried out to some extent during the self-evaluation period; however, the nurse should spend a little time each day comparing her own written records with those of her colleagues.

The nursing objectives are quite simple to follow and the reader has in many instances already been provided with criteria for assessment. This section on the concurrent nursing audit is concluded by identifying the basic objectives of the nurse within the framework of the nursing process:

Nursing objectives

● To identify initial patient problems on admission and construct interim care for solving or abating them.

● To establish a working relationship with the patient so that nurse and patient can function as a team.

● To document an accurate nurse's impression of the patient's relevant background and presentation.

● To produce a record of interview complementary to the nurse's impression so that a full profile is complete.

● To identify the areas of need experienced or presented by the patient in company with that patient.

● To identify the short- and long-term objectives related to the problem in the company of the patient.

● To construct a care programme relative to the satisfaction of the patient's needs and complementary to the medical programme being provided (including all other paramedical programmes being used by the patients for their recovery).

● To evaluate the effectiveness of the care plans and the care provided, including suitability and appropriateness.

● To involve the patient in every step of the process, seeking his advice and ideas and becoming familiar with his fears so that he becomes involved in his own care.

● To involve, where possible, the patient's family, friends and visitors in the production of the plans and the delivery of the care.

● To maintain quality of care provided and ensure that the care plans are adhered to.

● To evaluate the nurse's own performance at regular intervals to ensure that she has done the best for her patient within the limitations of the clinical area in which she has to work.

PATIENT PROGRESS

The second element of evaluation to be considered is that which uses the patient's progress as its criteria for assessment. As Richards and Lambert (1987) point out, this includes the patient's own evaluation of his care in conjunction with that of the nurses in an attempt to gain a more objective understanding of what is taking place. It is a commonly held belief that the only form of evaluation in nursing is that of the patient's progress through his illness in relation to the nursing he receives. As already shown, this is not strictly true, although it remains probably the most important of the areas in which evaluative procedure is employed.

In a series of articles, Boylan (1982) pointed out that, very often, patients leave hospital having recovered from their illnesses despite nurses rather than because of them. This theory carries considerable credence in some departments of psychiatry where patients are admitted with social problems over which the nurse has absolutely no control, where personal difficulties are never disclosed, and psychiatric symptoms never recognised as such. It is therefore necessary to be extremely careful, when evaluating patient progress, to ensure that outcomes which are beneficial to the patient are not automatically attributed to the direct actions of the nurse. This can only be done if the nurse is critical of what she does and has a clear understanding of the desired effects of the care she provides. This is achieved in part through her own professional education, and in part through her interactions with the patient himself who should provide her with information related to how he sees her care and what significance it has for him. Because of this, much of the evaluation procedure will centre around the patient's appreciation of how he sees himself progressing through his illness, as opposed to the nurse's observations, although of course these still remain of great importance. This evaluation procedure thus differs from that used in general nursing where very often the criteria for evaluation are the physical manifestations of illness.

When evaluating patient progress, then, the following areas must be included:

- date of evaluation
- behaviour to be evaluated
- patient's needs
- short-term objectives
- long-term objectives
- patient involvement, including that of relatives or friends
- modification of care plans
- the effectiveness of care provided
- the appropriateness of care provided
- the quality of care provided.

The effectiveness, appropriateness and quality of the care provided has already been discussed in this chapter, but it is worth stressing once more that the nurse must always seek the advice of the patient as to whether or not she is right in her assessment of her own actions.

DATE OF EVALUATION

The process of evaluation is taking place all the time; it is not something which should be restricted to certain moments. When people are getting ready to go out in the evening the final evaluation of their preparation may well be a glance in the mirror before leaving, but prior to that assessment or evaluation the procedure may well have been conducted a hundred times. Why do they wash their hair, take a shower, put different clothing on, clean their teeth, have a shave, have something to eat and drink, or wear after-shave or perfume? The answer is simple, they measure their existing state against that which they desire themselves to be in when they go out. They are aiming for their own personal perfection. The comparisons made are many and varied but all are types of evaluation or reassessment.

For the nurse working on a psychiatric ward

the same principle applies. She should be critical, appraise all the actions and observations made during her spell of duty in relation to what she already knows about her patients, and draw the necessary conclusions from them. This last point is important; nurses should always strive to understand the significance of their observations, otherwise they are simply observers and will have little or no control over what takes place. Once these observations have been made and analysed they must be recorded if necessary, and the use of SOAP notes (see Ch. 7) will facilitate following this phase of the procedure.

As well as this continuous evaluation there is the more formal approach required by the nursing process. The objectives set for the patient must have a time limit written into them. When that time limit expires, the evaluation of the patient's progress should be made in relation to the care given. In certain instances, it may not be possible to evaluate on the day designated, but the nurse must try and carry out the process at the prescribed time whenever possible to avoid unsuitable objectives being used as the guidelines for care. The evaluation is thus a two-fold affair consisting of:

1. continuous assessment of the patient's progress
2. formal evaluation of progress in relation to the care given at set times stipulated in the objective statements.

BEHAVIOUR TO BE EVALUATED

The behaviour to be evaluated will obviously largely depend on the patient himself, his problems, needs and personal environment. Most of this information will already have been synthesised and used in the production of the patient's objectives; however, the situation, though having many constant factors, is a fluid one, subject to constant change. A flexible approach is therefore necessary, and there are two evaluation areas where this flexibility should be exercised.

1. *Continuous (or general) assessment* – continuous monitoring of behaviour related to the short-

term objectives, changing patterns in presentation, alterations in the patient's personal circumstances (both social and physical), and information which might necessitate the modification of care objectives.

   2. *Formal (or projected) evaluation* – information related specifically to the expected outcomes of the care given which may require care plan modification and information specific to the long-term objectives.

For example, if a patient has been assessed during his initial stages of admission as having the nursing diagnosis, 'Is unable to dress because he cannot grasp buttons', and is given the long-term objective, 'Will be able to dress himself', and the short-term objective, 'Will be able to remove his pyjamas', the following might be observed during the first stage of continuous assessment:

1. Does not seem to understand what is required of him.
2. Complains of pain.
3. Seems disorientated in time and place.
4. Becomes agitated when approached.
5. Refuses to rise.
6. Has no difficulty in removing pyjamas but will not be helped to dress.
7. Can dress himself quite easily.
8. Is incontinent of urine and therefore has to be helped from his soiled clothes.

In some of these instances it will be necessary simply to modify the nursing care provided so that the short-term objective can still be achieved, e.g. as in 1, 2, 3, 4, 5 and 6 above; in others, the projected assessment may have to be altered because a higher priority need has been isolated, e.g. as in 8 and 2; and it may be that both the short- and long-term objectives will have to be modified, e.g. as in 2, 7, 6 and 3. The important point here is the inter-relatedness of the two evaluative areas. The general or continuous assessment feeds vital information to the projected assessment, thus producing care which is appropriate and consistent with the reality of the situation as is exists now, not as it was on admission. It is also perhaps worth mentioning that other influences too are monitored during the general presentation, for example the effects of:

- medically prescribed care
- para-medical intervention
- care prescribed by external agencies (in the case of patients receiving long-term care from other specialists).

These areas do not have significance for the projected evaluation as these are related solely to the nursing care. They are, however, of great importance because they constitute part of the overall scheme of care and will, therefore, have some effect on the patient and, indirectly, on his ability to respond to his nursing care. A good example of this is a patient who is receiving care related to his ability to converse and mix with other people, but who is receiving large doses of major tranquillisers. If the medication reduces his ability to communicate with others because it interferes with his level of consciousness, that information should be passed to the medical staff so that the doses can be reduced. Whilst this reduction is taking effect, however, the short-term objective may have to be reduced accordingly to accommodate the change in his ability; alternatively, the use of an expressive objective may be more appropriate. Hence, the continuous assessment feeds information both to the medical staff and to those responsible for the projected evaluation of the nursing process for the patient. The changes isolated are part of the patient's changing pattern of needs, even though those changes may themselves have been created by the health care team.

PATIENT'S NEEDS

We have already seen how the patient's needs can be changed by both external and internal influences. In many cases, the patient retains the same needs but either gains further ones because the initial ones are not satisfied, or others come to light which were not apparent at the production of the profile. The nurse must be prepared to adapt her activities to suit the particular requirement of the individual patient, and if necessary, to do so before the formal projected evaluation takes place. If a priority need is identified, the patient could well die if something is not done immediately; waiting till the end of the week will be too late. It may also be the case that during the continuous assessment the nurse realises that several of the patient's needs are being satisfied by the attention being paid to one particular need; she will therefore modify the care plan accordingly at the formal session so that unnecessary care is not offered to the patient.

Suppose, for example, that the following areas of need are identified by the nurse in a patient experiencing an excessively overactive phase of his presentation:

● the physical needs of eating, drinking, elimination and rest
● the psychosocial needs for deserved praise, communication, security and companionship.

Nursing care is provided for eating, drinking, resting, communication and companionship. During her continuous assessment, the nurse observes that the need for companionship is met by the care offered for communication purposes and that the need for rest can also be satisfied when this communication is of good quality. The companionship need is also met as the patient begins to eat and drink in the company of others. Thus, at the projected evaluation stage she concludes that care for the needs of rest and companionship, eating and drinking are all being catered for by the care delivered for satisfying communication needs. She is able to reduce the amount of care that is performed. By doing this she also creates time to offer care for deserved praise and security, having established that the need for elimination is already being met by the patient himself. In time, she may recognize duplication in these areas also and adjust the care plan accordingly.

SHORT-TERM OBJECTIVES

The short-term objectives are those small, easily attainable steps the patient is asked to achieve in his attempt to regain independence. In sequence,

these small steps will take him to the final or long-term objective. The short-term objective is evaluated both during the continuous assessment stage and at the formal projected evaluation stage. One of the elements of care plan modification is close scrutiny of the short-term objectives in comparison to the patient's behaviour. Certain questions should be asked:

1. Does the patient's behaviour match that outlined by the objective?

If the answer to this question is 'yes', then three other questions should be asked.

2. (i)   How soon did he achieve this objective?
    (ii) What is the next objective to be?
    (iii) If the objective was of an expressive nature how did the patient attempt to produce a result?

If the answer to question (1) is 'no' then several other questions must be asked.

3. (i)   Was the objective too difficult to achieve?
    (ii) Was the time allowed sufficient for the expected improvement?
    (iii) Should the quantifiable element in the objective be reduced, i.e. from two hours to one hour, from 1 kg to 0.5 kg etc?
    (iv) Was the expressive nature of the objective too difficult for the patient to understand, and was he ever given the opportunity to carry it out or practise it?
    (v)   Should anything be added to the objective to make it more realistic, e.g. in the company of a member of staff, etc?
    (vi) Is the objective really appropriate to the patient's need? If not, a new set of objectives should be found.

There are more questions that could be asked but these will centre around the individual nature of the objective, the patient and his care. Obviously, if the objective is to be of any value to the patient, what he is expected to do to achieve it must be within his capabilities and consistent with his eventual or long-term objective. Nurses must be prepared to change objectives, to re-word them or simply scrap them if they do not fit the bill. This activity should be carried out at the projected evaluation stage, but there is no reason why the responsible nurse cannot change the objectives during the continuous assessment phase. In doing so, however, she must ensure that all involved parties are aware of her actions and, in particular, that the patient has been consulted beforehand and understands the implications of the change. The patient may even ask for a change to be made, and this too must be given consideration and discussed with him.

The patient's progress in the nursing process is gauged by his ability to achieve his objectives, especially if he sets them himself. It is, therefore, of extreme importance that when nurses evaluate the short-term objective and compare it with the patient's behaviour the two should match perfectly. If the patient has not quite reached the expected behaviour, then he has not achieved his objective and it is pointless asking him to try to achieve the next one in the sequence. His care will become a deception. He will know this even if the nursing staff involved do not recognise it. He will cease to gain confidence in his own ability and may deteriorate because he does not see himself improving. In this situation, the nurse will not be able to reassure him by pointing to his past successes because he will not recognise them as such. Thus, one of the principal methods of applying psychiatric first aid will be denied the nurse in her attempt to lift the patient's flagging morale. Even if the patient is deceived into thinking that he is doing better than he really is by a nurse who desperately wants him to succeed for both his sake and hers, in the long run he is bound to recognise that all is not as well as he thought. One of the main objectives of the nursing process itself is to help the patient deal with his own problems. If the nurse tells a patient that he is capable of handling his life situation sufficiently well to be able to leave the hospital, and he then finds that he is still as incapable as when he was first admitted, the shock could be enough to irrevocably impede any future hopes of rehabilitation. The nurse has a duty to her patient to evaluate his progress in relation to his objectives in an honest and critical way. She will do neither herself nor her patient any good by hiding the truth.

LONG-TERM OBJECTIVES

Each of the major problem areas will have a long-term objective attached to it. These objectives outline the behaviour expected of the patient in each area when his care is complete. They need not necessarily coincide with his discharge from hospital, but may be achieved before he leaves or afterwards under the supervision of the community psychiatric nurse. The patient's long-term objectives are evaluated at the projected evaluation stage in the light of whether or not the short-term objectives are being reached or not. It is unusual for them to be changed with the same regularity as their short-term counterparts but they may be changed in the following situations:

• If a patient is recognised as having little or no potential in a particular problem area. This is often the case in the care of the elderly mentally ill where the patient's physical deterioration may interfere with his ability to carry out the most basic of tasks. The initial long-term objective may well be constituted before the patient's real condition is apparent. In this situation the long-term objective will have to be reduced considerably.

• If a patient is reaching his short-term objectives with ease, a greater potential is recognised. Certainly, in the medium long-stay areas this often becomes the case when patients suddenly regain forgotten or ill-used abilities and their motivation is rekindled. In this situation it will be necessary to increase the long-term objective.

• If a patient achieves a long-term objective within a very short space of time displaying no real need in that particular area at all. In this case the objective is simply regarded as achieved and the nurse can seek some other areas of maladaption. It may well be that this response to the clinical situation denotes early return to the community for the patient. This is sometimes the case in the acute areas, although it is not strictly limited to one clinical area. Elderly, mentally ill patients on their first admission often make dramatic improvements when confronted with new approaches to solving their problems.

PATIENT INVOLVEMENT

There are many ways in which the patient can be involved in the evaluation of his own progress. In some instances, of course, and perhaps in the early stages of hospitalisation, it may not be possible because the psychiatric symptoms are too severe for some patients to become totally involved in this activity. It should be one of the nurse's major objectives to get the patient to assess his own behaviour and try to promote an awareness of his effect on his own environment.

Where possible, relatives and friends should also be included as they have a far greater understanding of the way patients react to circumstances in their lives and can more accurately assess any change that is taking place (Shields 1985). By the same token, if modification is to take place in the care offered, relatives and friends should also be consulted about the part they can play in making it more realistic for the patient.

If the objectives are clearly laid out they should be easy enough for the patient to follow. The nurse may feel, through her observations during the continuous assessment phase, that a patient is quite happy with his progress or is managing to cope with the activities taking place. During the projected evaluation, however, he may well disclose fears and apprehensions which will necessitate changes being made in the objectives set. Sitting down at regular intervals and discussing the care offered and its effect on the patient with the patient himself will serve two purposes.

1. It will make him feel that he really does matter and that his opinion has meaning and importance.
2. It will keep the nurse informed as to the correct aspects of the patient's responses to the care situation.

However, informal discussions may not always be enough. Some patients find it difficult to assess themselves and need guidelines or structured questions to help them. Questionnaires or action criteria sheets can be produced with the patient's help to help them plot their progress. Personal effectiveness is a good example of this system. Many psychiatric patients have difficulty relating to others. Their effectiveness in terms of their own problem solving can often be directly related to their effectiveness in dealing with those around them (Harden et al 1986). If the patient is given a boxed sheet, headed with those areas of social skills which he finds most difficult to cope with, and is requested to place ticks in the appropriate boxes as he deals with them more effectively, e.g. eye contact, loudness of voice, sitting position, etc, he will have an ongoing record of his own activities. This written record can be assessed and analysed by the nurse and patient together and used as a self-evaluation tool for the patient. Self-charting or plotting is the best aid to self-evaluation for those patients who have difficulty abstracting events and experiences from their own life situation. However, other methods that might be employed are:

- Asking the patient to keep a form of diary related to specific situations or types of nursing intervention.
- Getting the patient to reward himself in some small way if the daily events go well.
- Asking the patient to test himself in certain difficult situations to see how he feels either during or on completion of the task.
- Always making the patient's objectives available to him so that he has a constant check of what he is expecting to achieve.
- Teaching the patient to be aware of areas related to his problems so that he can assess their influence and if possible do something about them.
- Helping the patient to be critical of his own actions and also to accept constructive criticisms from others.
- Being available to the patient so that he can discuss unforeseen changes in his environment or

appreciation of it. If the responsible nurse is not going to be available she should delegate a replacement and inform the patient of this, introducing the stand-in nurse when possible.

The majority of these self-evaluation techniques and methods require that the patient accept responsibility for his own actions. In most situations, the method will have to be explained fully so that the patient is aware of his own commitment and knows how to transfer or communicate the necessary information to the appropriate nurse or team. There are, of course, always going to be those patients who already have all the answers, those that are far too critical of themselves and those who are simply not prepared to accept any responsibility at all. In these cases, the nurse has to use her personal skills to help the patient get the most out of his evaluation sessions. This may involve increasing or decreasing her personal contact with him and, in most cases, will involve the use of considerable tact, patience and judgement. It must be remembered that psychiatric nursing is all about teaching, and if, at the end of a patient's contact with a nurse, he has learnt something of the art of self-evaluation he will have learnt a great deal and thus improved the quality of his hospitalisation (Shields & Morrison 1988).

CARE PLAN MODIFICATION

So far, we have discussed those elements of the evaluative process which are probably the most difficult to carry out. This is because in most instances they are often hypothetical and are greatly influenced by subjective thought. Furthermore, they do not always necessitate an active response to the conclusions the nurse comes to. It is often a case more of re-thinking rather than of re-doing, and with nothing concrete on which to base those thoughts, change or improvement in care can be extremely difficult.

The modification of the care plan by comparison between the previous and the present situation is a much easier exercise. The plan is a written document containing basic information derived from careful observation, assessment and professional knowledge. If the care plan has been kept simple, as has been suggested, the comparison process is carried out by asking three basic questions during the projected evaluation session:

1. Has the patient's nursing diagnosis changed in any way? If so, what is the new diagnosis? The patient's needs may remain unaltered but the level of competency in his methods of satisfaction may have improved or deteriorated.

2. Are the objectives for care still appropriate to the patient's level of progress, i.e. has he reached them or not?

3. Has the correct nursing care been provided that will link the need with the objective?

To illustrate how these questions are applied to the clinical situation the case study from the previous chapters will be used. The three areas of the plan will be examined in relation to new information. What takes place is the activity that should occur between the responsible nursing staff at the projected evaluation session. The dates of these sessions are determined by the objective achievement dates placed on the care plan. Such sessions will involve a team approach even if the team system does not actually exist on the ward. This means that the senior nurse will meet with either members of the nursing staff involved in the patient's care or allocated nurses, to evaluate the plan. Where the team system functions, this responsibility rests with the primary nurse on the team, who discusses the evaluation with all other available team members.

CASE STUDY: JULIE DAWSON

In effect, it has already been shown how the projected evaluation of Julie's care plan might take place by producing both an initial and an on-going outline. However, assuming that this is the 8th July 1991, the review date for Julie's on-going care plan (Fig. 6.2), it will be evaluated accordingly (care plan; see Fig. 8.1). The following is a summary of Julie's progress notes for her second week of admission.

Julie has made little progress in her communication with either fellow patients or assigned nursing staff. She will identify them only by names she has given them herself and sees them as nuns rather than nurses. She has been unable to discuss her feelings with them and manages to hold only stilted conversation. She still prefers the sanctuary of her own room but has managed to achieve her objectives (3) and (6). Her concentration appears very poor and she has little interest in current affairs or the realities of her environment. Her personal hygiene has improved a little but she will accept little responsibility for bathing or washing. Her parents have visited her on three occasions during the week and have become involved in some aspects of her care, in particular those centring around ward excursions and conversations. Both are prepared to become more involved if the need should arise or if the nursing staff can find ways to use their special relationship.

Julie's general presentation remains little changed, although there is some reduction in the amount of delusional activity perceived by the nursing staff. Julie herself will not discuss her thoughts or feelings, so much of the clinical information is still derived from observation of purely overt behaviour. Objectives (2), (4) and (5) have not been achieved though she has made some progress towards all three. Objective (4) needs to be altered to reflect the progress she has made, possibly converting from an expressive mode to a behavioural one, or altering the nature of the expressive component. It must be noted that she is sleeping well, at present an average of at least six hours per day, and that she is maintaining an acceptable fluid balance. One consequence of her tendency to lie in bed for long periods is that she has been incontinent of urine on two separate occasions. No breakdown of pressure areas.

Question One

- Has Julie's nursing diagnosis changed in any way?

Answer

- Yes – in areas (3) and (6).
- No – in areas (2), (4) and (5).
- Despite all new information and the difficulty of the urinary incontinence, no other problems have priority over the existing ones. Any new difficulties can be overcome by utilising existing nursing intervention.

What are the new diagnoses in areas (3) and (6)?

(3) Will only leave her room for two minutes at each excursion time.
(6) Will not eat meals, only small snacks at refreshment times.

Question Two

- Are the objectives still appropriate?

Answer

- Yes – in areas (2) and (5).
- No – in areas (3), (4) and (6).

New objectives are:

(3) Extend excursion time to ten minutes, and all meal and refreshment times.
(4) Will discuss a magazine with her parents each evening.
(6) Will sit at a meal table during meal times.

Question Three

- Has the correct nursing care been provided?

Answer

- Yes – but changes will be necessary as the objectives have been altered.

Review of appropriate nursing intervention

(2) To continue as before except that rota will contain daily allocations for conversations. Nurses to start to work on a theme taken from the discussion book. Reduce contact to nurse allocated for discussion.
(3) To continue as before but increase times.
(4) Nurses to liaise with parents about progress made and log items discussed.
(5) To continue as before but Julie prefers evening bath.
(6) Nurse to stay with Julie at meal times and preferably discuss food whilst at the table. Do not force Julie to eat. Congratulate her if she should eat.

The only other question that must be asked is, 'When are these objectives to be achieved?' To allow a reasonable period to achieve success, all objectives should be reviewed again in one week's time. The evaluations are written on the care plan, indicating who did them, whether or not Julie was involved, and what steps are to be taken. Review dates are set and the evaluating nurse, usually the primary nurse, initials the care plan. The progress notes should contain an entry to the effect that an evaluation has taken place and any corresponding information should also be noted, i.e. the consequences of changes or possibly the rationale, though in most cases this will not be necessary because of the care plan entry. If problems are no longer apparent they are removed completely from the care plan, with a line through the entry, with the word 'Achieved' written in the evaluation section. The problem itself will retain its number, and should it re-appear at a later date and need to appear on the care plan again, it will resume this same coded number.

Julie's evaluated care plan (Care Plan 2) is shown in Figure 8.1, and her new care plan (Care Plan 3) in Figure 8.2. Care Plans 2 and 3 will remain in Julie's current folder until they are no longer being used, at which time they will be filed for future reference.

READER EXERCISE

In the same way that a summary of Julie Dawson's progress notes in the case study has been provided, a summary of Susan's case is given here for the benefit of the reader, in order to evaluate the care plan prepared in Chapter 5.

READER CASE STUDY: SUSAN

There has been a marked change in Susan's overall presentation since her hospitalisation began. She has become solitary and morose, and refuses to become involved in even the smallest of interactions with the nursing staff. She openly abuses the other patients on the ward and has come close to being struck by one particular young patient. She has become totally inactive and often complains bitterly that she is bored and wishes to go home. Despite this lack of exercise, and probably because she refuses all meals except fruit, she has lost a further 0.5 kg in weight. She does take a lot of fluids, however, and her analysis shows no abnormalities. Susan's attention to personal hygiene is practically non-existent and she has developed the habit of hiding her clothes in her room so that the nursing staff do not discuss them with her. Most of her time is spent reading pseudo-psychology books on dreams and phobias which she asked her mother to bring in for her. She refuses all attempts to occupy her in any other way. Her father has not visited for a week, but her mother sees her every evening and Susan has begun to talk with her. Unfortunately, these visits usually end in an argument and mother leaves in tears. She is reluctant to

discuss her daughter with the nursing staff and it is generally felt that she may well ask to take Susan home with her in the near future.

The only person for whom Susan has a pleasant word is her doctor, with whom she appears to have a reasonable relationship.

He has indicated that he approves of the nursing intervention and feels that he has nothing further to request of the staff at this point. Susan's physical appearance is deteriorating. She has greasy skin and lank hair and a strong smell of body odour.

Answer the questions from the evaluation section listed below and amend your care plan for Susan accordingly on Figure 8.3.

Question One

- Has Susan's nursing diagnosis changed in any way?

Answer

- Yes – in areas ...
- No – in areas ...

What is the new diagnosis?

Question Two

- Are the objectives still appropriate?

Answer

- Yes – in areas ...
- No – in areas ...

New objectives are:

Nursing interventions	Evaluations	Date	Nurse's initials
② a) Increase contact to all team members. b) Produce roster for nurse conversation. c) Ensure contact each time till contact acknowledged by Julie. d) Document discussed conversation content.	Team evaluation – Julie would not take part. Has not achieved objective. Alter intervention to increase concentration – ie reduce nursing numbers, select topics.	8/7/91	KW
③ a) Increase toilet time to 2 mins. b) Introduce to other patients. c) Offer a drink whilst on excursion. d) Offer congratulations if she stays out of her room for long periods of time.	Team evaluation – Julie would not take part. Objective achieved. Increase new objective time. Keep intervention as it is.	8/7/91	KW
④ a) Discuss making list at beginning of shift. b) State time to discuss list. c) Remind of list at regular times during the shift – ie ½ hourly at first. d) Try to get her to expand as to why items appear on the list.	Team evaluation – Julie limited involvement. Objective partially achieved. Change objective to fit progress to date.	8/7/91	KW
⑤ a) Encourage a basin wash before bath. b) If Julie requests a bath at any time. – agree. c) Try to suggest bath at same time each day to establish a routine. Ask Julie which time would be best.	Team evaluation – Julie not involved. Objective partially achieved. Julie likes a bath in the evening – alter to accommodate her wishes.	8/7/91	KW
⑥ a) Ensure that one of her excursions coincides with refreshment breaks. b) If possible leave her in the company of other patients and observe discreetly.	Team evaluation – Julie not involved. Objective achieved. Alter objective to increase her time at dining table – intervention to suit.	8/7/91	KW

Primary nurse: Karen Walters   Sheet number: 2

Fig. 8.1 Julie Dawson's evaluated care plan (Care Plan 2).

Question Three

● Has the correct nursing care been provided?

Answer

● Yes – in areas ...
● No – in areas ...

Review of appropriate nursing intervention

RETROSPECTIVE NURSING AUDIT

Retrospective nursing audit has no influence upon the care delivered to a patient while he is hospitalised and is therefore not responsible for improvements in the normal sense of the word. The consequences of this evaluation, however, are reflected in the standard of care provided for future generations of patients. It is also the main method of maintaining overall quality control and should be used to introduce new ideas in technology and improved methods of delivering nursing intervention.

Evaluation of this nature does not single out individual nursing actions but looks at nursing as both a complete and a complementary agent in the patient's progress. As long ago as 1960, Peplau showed how nurses' behaviour could have a direct bearing on the patient's perception of how to respond in given circumstances, even though the nurses may be unaware of their influence. The retrospective audit allows nurses to look back on their achievements and establish, in relation to the patients' progress notes, what those influencing factors could be and how they can be used to better effect in future interactions.

NURSING AUDIT GROUPS II

By far the best method of carrying out the retrospective audit is the audit group. It can be constituted from both senior and junior nursing staff, although senior staff are more likely to have the necessary skills to evaluate care, and be drawn from either a selection of wards in one nursing unit or similar types of wards. Representatives from nursing management and medical and paramedical staff could be invited to attend specific meetings to discuss the nurses' activities, as they have influenced them. The committee meets at regular intervals, perhaps once a month, and discusses one case at each meeting.

The information at their disposal is as follows:

● the patient's profile, including nurse's impression and interview
● the patient's progress notes
● discharge notes, both medical and nursing
● medical documentation
● paramedical records
● care plans
● all other relevant documentation.

The case is presented to the committee by the senior nurse of the team responsible for the patient's care. It is not necessary for minute investigation to take place, but a broad summary of events should be given. Points of discussion might include:

● Particular difficulties encountered in the nursing interview and how these were overcome.
● The use of external disciplines, family and relatives.
● The difficulties of hidden problem areas and how they were eventually made to surface.
● Problems of need identification.
● The influence of patient cooperation or non-cooperation.
● The success or failure of the nursing intervention and the team's thoughts on their activities.
● The suitability of the nursing intervention in relation to the patient's perception of his problem.
● Difficulties in introducing new ideas.
● Plans for discharge and community staff liaison.

Patient Care Plan

Patient name: ...*Julie Dawson*.........   Clinical area: *Bowthorpe Villa*..........

Date	Nursing diagnosis	Patient/nursing objectives	Review date
8/7/91	① Cannot relate her feelings to those around her. — unable to establish a relationship.	① Will discuss her feelings with the allocated nurse at least once during each shift period.	15/7/91
8/7/91	③ Will only leave her room for 2 minutes at each excursion time.	③ Extend excursion time to 10 minutes and all meals and refreshment times.	15/7/91
8/7/91	④ Cannot see any purpose in her real existence as she has nothing to do.	④ Will discuss a magazine with her parents when they visit her in the evenings.	15/7/91
8/7/91	⑤ Fails to wash herself, dress or groom.	⑤ Will take a daily bath.	15/7/91
8/7/91	⑥ Will not eat meals, only small snacks at refreshment times.	⑥ Will sit at meal table during meal times.	15/7/91

Fig. 8.2A   Julie Dawson's new care plan (Care Plan 3).

Nursing interventions	Evaluations	Date	Nurse's initials
② a) Reduce contact to allocated nurses. b) Discuss specific topics – take theme from book. c) Gradually bring conversation around to the way she feels – discuss anything she says about her feelings.			
③ a) Increase toileting times for as long as possible b) Invite her to sit with other patients. c) Offer a drink whilst on excursion. d) Congratulate long stays from room.			
④ a) Continue with list. b) Discuss developments with parents – ask them to report back about any progress – tell them not to push Julie into discussing magazine – give them support and show how to approach the task.			
⑤ a) Encourage a basin wash before bath. b) If Julie requests bath at any time agree. c) Suggest bath in evening.			
⑥ a) Nurse to stay with Julie at meal times. b) Discuss food at dining table. c) Do not force Julie to eat. d) Congratulate her if she eats.			

Primary nurse: Karen Walters   Sheet number: 3

Fig. 8.2B Julie Dawson's new care plan (Care Plan 3) (cont'd).

Patient Care Plan

Patient name: ....   Clinical area: ....

Date	Nursing diagnosis	Patient/nursing objectives	Review date

Fig. 8.3A   Reader exercise: Susan's care plan (for evaluation).   © Longman Group UK Limited 1992

Nursing interventions	Evaluation	Date	Nurse's initials

Primary nurse: ....

Sheet number: ....

Fig. 8.3B   Reader exercise: Susan's care plan (for evaluation) (cont'd).

© Longman Group UK Limited 1992

- Medical, paramedical and nursing continuity.
- The patient's impression of his hospitalisation.
- Prognosis in terms of whether or not the nursing staff have taught the patient enough about himself for him to be able to deal with similar pre-morbid circumstances in the future.
- The positive aspects of the overall programme that might have benefit for future care.

Discussion about these and any number of other problems or success areas would hinge around the total, and not the individual, intervention. This ensures a far more effective approach to the evaluative procedure. Having a representative group of this nature should ensure that the views and opinions of a broader section of the nursing community are heard. If only one person, either a nursing officer, care manager or a senior clinical specialist, were to carry out the audit, that person's influence could create too much bias in one area, thus reducing the nurse's scope and choice of alternatives. It is also worth considering whether nurse management should be responsible for care evaluation. Senior clinical staff are likely to have a better appreciation of the nature and style of contemporary psychiatric nursing, though this may not necessarily be the case with managerial staff whose work priorities may have altered as a consequence of their job.

Following the discussion, the group should draw some conclusions from the presentation, offering advice and making recommendations that might be of use to nurses when dealing with similar problems in the future. These conclusions are in turn distributed to the various wards so that all the nursing teams can benefit from the committee's work.

STANDARD CARE PLANS

After this group has met on several occasions, it is possible to look at common problems and circumstances that appear regularly for both the patient and the nurse. If a problem is usually dealt with effectively by the same means on each occasion, this could be regarded as a standard plan of action. Taking this to its logical conclusion, it is conceivable that standard care plans (Kurose et al 1981) could be produced for each of the major presenting conditions which contained problems and actions that conformed with a basic pattern of events. Information could be taken from the standard care plan, if it fitted the individual patient's condition, and incorporated into the nursing care plan. This would save both time and effort on the part of the patient and the nurse, and would offer the nurse a tried and trusted method of dealing with a particular problem. Of course, it would be foolish to suggest that this would be possible for the great mass of intricate problems that each individual patient identifies, but there are areas, even in psychiatry, which would benefit from this type of procedure. For example:

- the alcoholic patient suffering from the effects of delirium tremens
- the elderly patient who cannot eliminate
- the patient who cannot feed himself
- the patient who is antisocial
- the patient who wishes to discharge himself against medical and nursing advice.

These standard care plans will not themselves constitute the patient's on-going intervention programme, but could ensure that common problems are dealt with in the most effective way. This is maintaining quality. It must be remembered that just as all other areas should be open to scrutiny so too must the standard care plan; if used, it must be updated and reviewed to preserve its suitability. Standard care plans should not be used where there is any doubt about their effectiveness or appropriateness to the patient's requirements.

RESEARCH

The other task of the retrospective audit group should be to initiate, carry out and monitor small scale research, either independently or in collaboration with the nurse education department or research and development staff. Nurses should be able to prove, through research:

1. what they are doing
2. how they are doing it.

Care plans can themselves form the basis of a research project. Baradell (1990) uses client-centred consultation as a specific research design.

In the past, nurses have tended to rely far too heavily on the research of other disciplines for their information about health care (Aggleton & Chalmers 1986). Very often, this information is related to the needs of the nurse and her patients, but not always (Walsh & Ford 1989). Such research should be adapted and used by nurses to establish how circumstances are affected in a patient–nurse configuration. This means researching from a nursing angle, restating the case in nursing terms and rediscovering the implications of nursing actions. The audit group may well be faced with such questions as, How was this event influenced? What precipitated it? Why did it take place? and What were its consequences? – and they may not have the answers. It would be wrong of them in that situation simply to assume the answers. They must find out the real answers or they are failing in the basic task of a scientific and dynamic approach to their evaluation.

Areas that the audit group might decide to investigate include:

- the effects of team nursing on the patient's perception of his involvement in his own care
- the use of standard care plans
- the effectiveness of the nursing process documentation
- better methods of patient–nurse allocation
- the effectiveness of nursing personnel in certain set circumstances
- patient understanding of their hospitalisation
- the communication patterns that develop within the nursing process framework
- interdisciplinary activities
- quality control measuring techniques
- the standard of nursing care produced by the nursing process itself
- developing action research strategies for different types of objectives.

These are just a few examples of the areas that should be looked at by the nurse. There are many more, and they arise from the everyday activities of nurses who are bewildered by their successes or failures, or simply need to know why events take place in the way they do. Only through a better understanding of the interactions of people, places and events affected by the health care situation, can nurses hope to manipulate these variables to achieve the best possible result. Because the audit group has no executive powers, it will rely heavily on the commitment of those nurses working within the various departments for its work in research. This does not mean that in its recommendations the audit group cannot state the need for investigation – a basic human need.

SUMMARY

This chapter has been divided into three main areas: concurrent nursing audit, patient progress and retrospective nursing audit. The process of evaluation is a vital part of any scientific action, and so has been looked at in some depth and not only in relation to the modification of patient care plans. The nurse must be able to examine her actions in relation to her colleagues and her patients, and understand what part she has to play in the interactions between them. The concurrent nursing audit begins by the nurse examining her own actions and establishing her own strengths and weaknesses. She must be professional enough to accept that while the perfect nurse does not exist, through self-evaluation she can strive to become as close to that ideal as possible. She has to understand herself first before she can hope to understand others. Once she has made herself aware of this and has begun the long task of critical appraisal, she can move onto the next stage, that of evaluating the progress of others – in this case, the progress of her patients.

The patient always has a very clear picture of the nurse, even though at times is an incorrect image, and part of that picture is a confident, caring individual. The nurse can demonstrate her confidence and her care by helping the patient to decide upon his future activities. She does this through the simple process of evaluating his behaviour in relation to his expectations, and then teaching him how to either improve or modify one or both of them. She must do this with all the professional skill she can muster. This entails being constantly vigilant as to the quality of her interventions and of her decisions about her patient. Careful and enlightened evaluation is the key to the effectiveness of the care she provides.

Finally, when the patient has received the care that is his right, and left the hospital environment to test his ability elsewhere, the nurse must carry out the last stage of the evaluation procedure – that of retrospective nursing audit. She must go back over the whole programme and examine it once again for its flaws, for its successes and for the lessons it can teach her for her next patient contact. It is not a crime to make mistakes but it is a crime not to learn from them. A nurse who makes mistakes and does not learn from them is making a mould for herself which she will find very difficult to break. If she persists in this rigid approach to one area of her work it will begin to creep into other aspects of her work until eventually she becomes short sighted in her approach to patient care. It is almost inevitable that a cynical attitude will develop with a stereotyped approach to her

work; and her failure to change will hinder her ability to recognise patients' problems as individual difficulties unique to them alone because they themselves are unique. Her attitude may alienate her from the more flexible members of the nursing team and friction between them will be reflected in the day-to-day interactions. The consequences of this for effective patient–nurse activity could well be disastrous. If nursing in psychiatry is to achieve the level of excellence expected of professionals, then the team must function as such, not as frustrated individuals with neither trust nor confidence in each other. Only by working together and carrying out insightful evaluation of their effectiveness can a nursing team produce a standard of nursing care commensurate with their knowledge of human behaviour and their expectations of themselves as caring people. Think of it this way: if you were admitted to a hospital tomorrow what sort of nursing care would you want?

REFERENCES

Aggleton P, Chalmers H 1986 Nursing research, nursing theory and the nursing process. Journal of Advanced Nursing 11: 197–202

Baradell J G 1990 Client-centred case consultation and single-case research design: application to case management. Archives of Psychiatric Nursing 4(1): 12–17

Boylan A 1982 Nursing at the crossroads 2. The nursing process and the role of the registered nurse. Nursing Times 78(34): 1443–1444

Dietrich G 1978 Teaching psychiatric nursing in the classroom. Journal of Advanced Nursing 3: 525–534

Harden J, Hales R E et al 1986 In-patient participation in treatment programming: a preliminary report. General Hospital Psychiatry 8(4): 287–290

Kurose et al 1981 A standard care plan for alcoholics. American Journal of Nursing 81(6): 1001–1006

Lauri S 1982 Development of the nursing process through research. Journal of Advanced Nursing 7: 301–307

McFarlane Baroness of Llandaff, Casthedine G 1982 A

guide to the practice of nursing using the nursing process. C V Mosby, St Louis, p. 128

Peplau H 1960 Talking with patients. American Journal of Nursing 60: 964–966

Richards D A, Lambert P 1987 The nursing process: the effect on patient satisfaction with nursing care. Journal of Advanced Nursing 12(2): 559–562

Shields P J 1985 The consumers view of psychiatry. Hospital and Health Service Review 81: 117–119

Shields P J, Morrison P 1988 Consumer satisfaction on a psychiatric ward. Journal of Advanced Nursing 13: 396–400

Vogel N A 1988 Development and use of a nursing process audit instrument. Nursing Management 19(8): 71, 74, 76

Walsh M, Ford P 1989 Nursing rituals: research and rational actions. Heinemann Nursing, Oxford, pp. 150–155

Zimmer M J 1976 Quality assurance of outcomes of patient care. Nursing Clinics of North America 9(2): 305–315

SUGGESTED READING

Brar A 1989 Nursing audit: an evaluation of nursing care. Nursing Journal of India 80(10): 268–269

Hurst K, Dean A 1987 An investigation into nurses' perceptions of problem-solving in clinical practice. In: Hannah K J, Reimer M et al (eds) Clinical judgement and decision making: the future with nursing diagnosis. John Wiley & Sons, New York, pp. 409–411

Kasch C R, Knutson K 1986 The functional message behaviour inventory. Nurse Practitioner 11(6): 61–67

van Maanen H M 1984 Evaluation of nursing care: a multi-national perspective. In: Willis L D, Linwood M E (eds) Measuring the quality of care. Churchill Livingstone, Edinburgh

SECTION 2
Clinical approach

9

The nursing process in acute psychiatry

INTRODUCTION

The nurse involved in acute psychiatry very often has less time available to her to scientifically plan and deliver nursing interventions than she would do in other areas of the discipline. Furthermore, the knowledge base from which these interventions must be conceptualised tends to be much larger. The nurse may be faced with any number of possible alternatives when dealing with patients whose behaviour is often disruptive and at times alarming. Add to this the wide range of age differences, medical diagnoses and personality complications that may be present in the patient population at any one time, and the reader can begin to understand the problems facing the nurse as she attempts to provide effective nursing care.

In this chapter, a care study is examined in the context of these difficulties. Some indications of the time factor involved, staff communications and other patient commitments have also been included. The actual case work is carried out by a staff nurse who is the primary nurse for a group of four nurses, and the whole of the study will be viewed through her eyes. Allocation, roles and responsibilities will also play a part in the overall presentation.

The process discussed in the previous chapters of scientifically observing, assessing, planning, implementing and evaluating will be used, but some of the difficulties faced by the group, and in particular by the primary nurse, will be examined. It must be remembered that the approaches adopted by the group need not necessarily correspond to those the reader might use. What is important here are not the approaches themselves but the methods by which they are conceived, i.e. the workings of the nursing process.

PATIENT BACKGROUND

Raymond Smith was aged 19 and had been at university studying history for nearly a year when he came to the notice of his course tutor. Until that time he had been regarded as a relatively average individual who had a small group of friends, worked quite hard at his studies and was expected to do reasonably well if not outstandingly so. Little was known about his campus social life but no one had complained of his behaviour in any way and he was therefore unnoticed by the authorities. On the 25th May 1991, he was heard shouting in the student accommodation block where he resided, and despite numerous attempts to get him to calm down he refused to leave his room or unlock the door so that his friends could talk to him. The shouting continued and security staff came and unlocked his door. Raymond was totally naked and his room was in an appalling state of disarray, with broken glass littering the floor. The doctor and his personal tutor were sent for, and after they had spent nearly an hour with him he seemed much calmer and apologised profusely for his actions. No action was taken though the doctor suggested a further visit to his clinic in the morning. Raymond spent the night in the company of his friends and did not attend surgery the following day. Over the next few weeks he failed to attend lectures, did not produce assignment work and saw less and less of his close friends. When counselled by his tutor he exclaimed that he no longer had any desire to remain at university as it was boring.

His tutor became more concerned about his behaviour and once again decided to ask the doctor for advice. A meeting was arranged for the following day. That night Raymond was taken into custody by a police officer in the city after he was found swimming in the river at 3 o'clock in the morning. Whilst at the police station he became aggressive and abusive towards the police and a police surgeon visited him in his cell. The police surgeon could find no evidence of drug or alcohol abuse, but was struck by Raymond's obvious disturbed state of mind. He talked to himself continuously and it was with great effort on the doctor's part that he was able to hold a disjointed conversation with him. The main theme of the conversation was that someone or something had changed the inside of Raymond's head and was beginning to eat away at the rest of his body. He said that he felt no pain. A psychiatrist was called and it was mutually agreed by the two doctors that Raymond was suffering from a psychiatric reaction, accompanied by depersonalisation sensations, acute delusions of persecution and possible hallucination. His mood swings were quite dramatic, one minute quite calm and relaxed, the next both verbally and physically aggressive with no external precipitating causes. His main concern was that he should be left alone.

Raymond refused any form of medication and it was felt necessary to transfer him to the safety of an acute ward at the psychiatric hospital. He refused to be moved and despite the attention of the medical staff could not be persuaded. It was decided to place him on section two of the Mental Health Act 1983 enabling him to be admitted against his wishes and held for a period of 28 days for the basic purpose of assessment. In these unfortunate circumstances and in a borrowed set of clothing he was transported under police escort to the nearby hospital.

Preparations

The psychiatrist who had visited him in his police cell was not going to be responsible for him after his admission to hospital, so he phoned the appropriate colleagues who relayed the above information to the ward. Preparations were made for his arrival, and the sister on duty allocated Raymond to Staff Nurse Jenny Wright, the primary nurse for one of the three teams active on the ward. Only one other member of Nurse Wright's group was on duty that morning and she already had a busy case load to contend with. There were three other staff on duty excluding the sister; all were male, and if necessary Nurse Wright could call on them. She checked their allocations and discovered that one, in particular, might be made available if called upon in an emergency. He was approached and agreed to any necessary extra cross-group involvement. Next, Nurse Wright prepared the usual documentation and Raymond's bed, and awaited his arrival whilst attending to the five sets of care plans that she had allocated herself.

INITIAL DATA

When Raymond arrived on the ward he was accompanied by two police officers, his personal tutor, a friend from the university and a social worker. They were all shown into the interview room and, after a brief discussion with the sister, the case was formally handed over to Nurse Wright. The police left and Raymond seemed reasonably settled, though inquisitive as to his surroundings.

At this point, several decisions had to be made. Nurse Wright had been given the initial information about Raymond second-hand, from a doctor who had not attended the original interview, and now the picture presented did not tally with that data. She asked her third-year student to inform the doctor of Raymond's arrival and arranged for everyone to get a cup of tea. Next, after introducing herself as Jenny Wright, she decided to ask a few general questions of everyone present to get a clear picture of the situation. Several information sources were available to her:

- Raymond, the patient
- the personal tutor
- Raymond's friend
- the social worker.

Nurse Wright already had some preliminary information from the doctor. She asked questions about that information related to:

- how Raymond had arrived at the hospital
- why he felt he was in a hospital

- what circumstances had brought about his admission
- what were Raymond's wishes
- how could she help.

The replies she received from Raymond tended to indicate that the majority of her original data was correct, but the responses she received were rather tense and offhand.

- He did not know why he was in hospital.
- He was not aware that this was a hospital.
- He did not do anything wrong.
- He did not have anything wrong with him.
- He wanted to be left alone.
- He needed to see a doctor because something inside him was not quite here?

During this short interview, Jenny Wright realised that Raymond was a little afraid but she could not determine the exact reason for this. After 15 minutes she showed him his room, answered some general questions that he had, and initiated the customary admission documentation. The social worker and tutor left, and the third-year student remained with Raymond and his friend discussing his feelings. Until now all had gone reasonably well. Jenny Wright had made some observations on Raymond's behaviour; his responses to her, the questions he had asked, his general interest in himself and his surroundings and the small number of clinical symptoms that he presented. She was a little troubled that his behaviour did not correspond with that which she had anticipated but decided that if handled properly, with consideration and respect, a recurrence might be averted. The initial observations were recorded on the admission sheet and discussed with the sister.

Comments

This is a relatively straightforward situation: information about a patient to be admitted has resulted in some preconceived ideas about his presentation. Sometimes these ideas are ill-founded, sometimes not, but the nurse has to ensure that her own feelings do not interfere with her ability to be positive and objective in her approach towards the patient on his arrival. A very quick assessment of the situation determines the level of attention required, having prepared for alternatives before the patient arrives.

All information sources are utilised quickly and effectively to see if they have any relevant facts to add to the existing database. General discussion where possible with the patient elicits the essentials required to initiate immediate nursing intervention and becomes the first stage towards producing a nursing impression. The information is recorded and discussed with colleagues. The time spent with Raymond by the student will have to be discussed also, though at a later date. The initial entry in Raymond's progress notes centres only around a brief description of his admission circumstances and his formal status. (The legal documentation is attended to at the exact point of admission.)

Notice that a member of the team has been with Raymond since admission and this will continue for at least the remainder of the shift and probably longer.

The primary nurse now has the task of easing Raymond into the ward, helping him orientate himself, allowing him the opportunity to establish what is required of him without interfering with his autonomy, and at the same time finding out as much as possible about his ability to lead an independent existence. The first 24 hours of a patient's hospitalisation is a crucial period of time. If the transition from the outside environment to the ward is badly managed, it may have serious effects on the patient's ability to respond in a therapeutic fashion. All attempts to allow him to readjust at his own pace should be made.

INTERIM CARE PLAN

It was necessary for Jenny Wright to produce spontaneous nursing intervention on Raymond's arrival, but she now has the job of producing a interim care plan so that some degree of continuity can be established from the very beginning of his stay.

After completing her report and discussing her findings with the sister, Staff Nurse Wright went

back to Raymond's room. He had been seen by his doctor and the medical information was related to her. They discussed expected and actual behaviour, and it was decided not to initiate any form of drug therapy until a clear picture developed. The doctor told her that Raymond was possibly suffering auditory hallucinations and depersonalisation feelings. Raymond was convinced something terrible was happening to his body, yet did not seem too concerned about it. He was prepared to accept any treatment the doctor prescribed but had said it really was not necessary.

The initial medical interview had provided Jenny Wright with little information. She needed to establish what Raymond's immediate needs were and construct some form of nursing intervention to meet them. She spent the next half hour in the company of Raymond and his friend talking about anything he wanted, but asking the occasional question of her own. They walked around the ward meeting several other patients and staff members. Jenny Wright observed his comments, his questions, his attitudes, his general approach and his behaviour towards his environment and the people he met in it. They discussed the wards, her job and her function as his nurse. Eventually, they were joined by the student nurse and she was able to discuss what had happened in the staff nurse's absence. Raymond and his friend were left alone for a while and the two nurses went to the nursing station to discuss their observations. They split their observations into three areas:

1. *Physiological*

   • He appeared very tired and stated he had not slept for two nights.
   • He was not wearing his own clothes. He was quite annoyed about this fact.
   • He was hungry but refused any food.
   • He was reasonably active.
   • He seemed a little over-responsive to sudden noises.
   • Personal hygiene appeared neglected, especially his hair.

2. *Psychological*

   • He described quite frightening apparent

hallucinatory sensations/perceptions, yet was almost indifferent towards them.

- He went to great lengths to justify his behaviour.
- He asked lots of questions about whether or not he could leave, what he would do and his personal rights.

3. *Sociological*

- He had to be drawn into conversation, and usually responded in an abrasive manner.
- He felt comfortable in the presence of his friend but had reacted quite noisily to the doctor.
- He had not initiated any conversation with anyone other than those who had been introduced to him.
- He was a difficult man to talk to and became easily antagonised.

Their general impression was that at times Raymond appeared to be a little disorientated, found difficulty separating hallucinatory activity from fact, became abrasive because he felt threatened and was most comfortable in the company of his friend whom he trusted. He appeared to have accepted both Jenny Wright and Carol Dean, the student, but only tentatively.

They isolated his immediate needs as:

- sleep
- freedom from fear
- orientation
- personal hygiene.

They converted those assessments into the following nursing diagnoses (Fig. 9.1):

1. *Orientation.* Cannot discriminate between reality and sensory deception.
2. *Freedom from fear.* Does not feel safe in the ward environment and is abrasive towards others.
3. *Sleep.* No sleep for at least the last 48 hours.
4. *Personal hygiene.* Has body odour, greasy hair.

These diagnoses were written on the care plan and Jenny Wright went and discussed them with Raymond. He denied the existence of any hallucinatory activity, but did admit that he felt uncomfortable, and wanted to leave. The last two diagnoses he was non-committal about. He said he did not really care about anything but agreed to discuss possible objectives. With the aid of his friend a contract was agreed, and the following objectives seemed to be the most appropriate for the situation.

IMMEDIATE OBJECTIVES (SHORT-TERM)

1. To discuss with allocated nurse things he cannot explain. (Expressive)
2. To describe how he feels in the company of others. (Expressive)
3. To be in bed by 2100 hours. (Behavioural)
4. To have a bath/wash his hair before bed. (Behavioural)

The two nurses once again conferred. They looked at their existing quota of patients, at the times they were most busy and at the special therapy area they had to manage, and then decided upon their nursing intervention for Raymond. They had also to consider the involvement of the night staff who were not allocated to any nursing team but who were responsible to each of them.

NURSING INTERVENTION

1. *Orientation*

- Encourage Raymond to keep a diary of his experiences.
- Discuss these at least once every hour.
- Do not interrupt him speaking.
- Spend at least 5 minutes with him if he approaches you.

2. *Freedom from fear*

- Only allocated nurse to approach him.
- Do not reinforce abrasive behaviour.

3. *Sleep*

- Night staff to be introduced by allocated nurse.

- Ensure restful environment from 2045 hours (in own room).

4. *Personal hygiene*

- All toilet requisites to be made available by 2000 hours.
- Encourage to have a bath.
- Praise appearance afterwards.

The information and instructions were also discussed with Raymond, though he could not see the justification for some of the areas covered. He was not shown the actual nursing intervention as written down on the care plan, but the basis of it was outlined to him. He was neither in agreement nor disagreement, but merely stated that it seemed 'OK'. The above information was then transferred to the care plan (Fig. 9.1).

Comments

Several factors are worth mentioning here. Firstly, the use of the diary for Raymond: Jenny Wright has used his academic background to get him involved in his own treatment situation. Whether it works will depend largely on the nurse's approach to its contents.

Secondly, only allocated nurses, i.e. those on Jenny Wright's team, will nurse Raymond. That does not mean that other nurses on the ward ignore him; they must be made aware of his problems and his nursing intervention so that they can respond accordingly if he should approach them. However, the idea here is that Raymond learns to trust a certain group of nurses rather than the whole nursing team. Eventually, he should be able to interact with all the ward staff, but it is too much to expect him to be able to do this immediately, especially with the added difficulty of his psychiatric symptomatology.

Thirdly, the night staff involvement and co-operation is very important. They must continue the care regime throughout the twilight hours but may have many more commitments on the ward. It is essential that Jenny Wright does not allocate night staff too much specialist care and she must check the amount of specific intervention already required of them. Her other major consideration in this area is that she does not ask them to do something complicated or intricate without first discussing it with them to see if they are able to comply. In this instance, giving a patient a bath and settling him down early in the evening, should not present too many problems. However, their responses and observations the following morning may well indicate a change in the care plan interventions.

Finally, the review dates for each of the nursing diagnoses are different. As Raymond's presentation unfolds, the objectives may need to be altered or they may be achieved quite quickly, thus alleviating the problem. The experienced nurse must show skill in selecting a suitable time for the achievement of each objective, and it could be argued that setting a review date slightly later than necessary is more suitable than setting one too early. In this case, Jenny Wright decided that each of her set objectives should show some degree of attainment within the first week. Interim care plans that have review dates two or three weeks later are perhaps asking too much of the nurse's observational and planning ability; nor do they take into consideration the changing pattern of the patient's behaviour following admission/transfer. This particular interim care plan has been designed with only two hours observation material as its basis. Over the next few days much may arise to change that original interpretation.

The initial interim plan must cater for the immediate needs of the patient and try to overcome some of the trauma caused by hospital admission. Consideration of long-term objectives may form only a minor part of the initial programme.

At lunch, Raymond's friend left and promised to return later that afternoon. Jenny Wright asked him a few questions concerning Raymond's usual behaviour, friends and hobbies, and made a note in the progress notes of the relevant data. Raymond declined food and his psychiatric symptomatology made it difficult to communicate with him.

On staff handover, a third member of the team came on duty, EN Paul Williams, replacing the student, Carol Dean. Jenny Wright handed over the care plan to Paul and outlined its major points to the other members of the team. Two other patients had been admitted that morning and all the team members made notes about their respective interim care plans as presented by the primary nurses. The sister then handed over the general data to the ward teams, and the primary nurses allocated the afternoon's patients to their teams. This handover was staggered as it was impossible for all the teams to be present at any one time. The most important part of the handover involved the three primary nurses and the sister.

AFTERNOON PRESENTATION

During the afternoon, Raymond's behaviour changed markedly. He was threatening and aggressive towards Paul Williams who was assigned to his care plan. The small headway that Jenny Wright had made in the morning did not seem to have any effect, and Raymond would not respond at all to any of the various approaches adopted by the team. Sister's advice was sought but she felt that they should continue as outlined on the care plan. Raymond remained in his room, shouting and gesticulating at anyone who approached. At 1600 hours when his friend returned he was much the same towards him. The doctor decided that some form of drug therapy should be initiated and prescribed a regime of major tranquillisers. Much to everyone's surprise, Raymond took the medication and seemed quite pleased to do so. This allowed EN Williams the opportunity to sit and talk to him and his friend, and in a short while the whole situation appeared to have calmed down. The doctor had spoken to Raymond's father on the telephone who had said he would be visiting the next day as he and his wife had a long way to travel. Jenny Wright was able to gain some insight into Raymond's background from the doctor's notes.

- Raymond had always been a quiet boy, interested more in academic than in physical pursuits.

- He did not have many close friends though he was reasonably popular at school.
- His main hobby appeared to be reading.
- He and his father had always had a close relationship, and his father had not wanted him to go to a university that was so far away from home.
- His father had noticed a change in him since he had been at university.
- His father also felt that Raymond was afraid of being at university but he could not be more specific about his feelings.
- Raymond's only sister, who was older than him, was also very close to him but she was married and had not seen much of him for the last 2 years.

Obviously, a considerable amount of the data would have to be looked at in Raymond's company when his parents arrived, but it did give the team something to begin with.

Comments

Data gathered from close relatives cannot always be regarded as absolute truth, because they are subjectively involved with the patient. It often gives a very accurate description of the way they feel about the individual but should always be verified by discussing it with the patient himself. In any case, such data gives the nurse something relevant to talk to the patient about, making their interactions more specific to him.

FIRST NIGHT

Raymond had a poor night. He got on well with the night staff, who were able to talk quite freely to him. Unfortunately, Raymond wanted to talk all night and, although this was good from the point of view of establishing a rapport and investigating his feelings, it meant that he had gone for a further period without real sleep. He was quite disturbed, and much of what he said was interrupted by his perceptional disturbances. It was noted that he felt more relaxed in the company of female staff and became restless and antagonistic towards male staff. He did have a

Patient Care Plan

Patient name: _Raymond Smith_ ....   Clinical area: _Bowthorpe Villa_ ....

Date	Nursing diagnosis	Patient/nursing objectives	Review date
1/6/91	① Cannot distinguish between reality and sensory deception.	① Discuss with allocated nurse things he cannot explain.	3/6/91
1/6/91	② Does not feel safe in the ward environment and is abrasive towards others.	② To describe how he feels in the company of others.	7/6/91
1/6/91	③ No sleep for at least 24 hours.	③ To be in bed by 2100 hrs.	3/6/91
1/6/91	④ Has body odour / greasy hair.	④ Have a bath / wash hair before retiring for bed.	2/6/91

Fig. 9.1A   Raymond Smith's interim care plan.

bath and was finished by 2300 hours; despite appearing extremely tired, he spent little time actually in bed and no time at all asleep. He was beginning to look quite drawn in the face and found it difficult to maintain his concentration for more than a limited period of time.

At the handover in the morning Raymond refused to leave the nursing station, so much of the information about other patients was passed on whilst the staff walked around the ward. Jenny Wright handed the care plan for Raymond to EN Paul Williams, but it was soon clear that

Primary nurse: _Jenny Wright_		Sheet number: _1_	
Nursing interventions	Evaluations	Date	Nurse's initials
① a) To encourage Raymond to keep a diary of his experiences. b) Nurses to discuss at least once a day. c) Do not interrupt him when he is speaking. d) Spend at least 5 minutes with him if he approaches you.			
② a) Only allocated nurse to discuss this topic with him. b) Try to catch him after he has had an encounter with someone else.			
③ a) Night staff to be introduced by allocated nurse. b) Ensure rest environment from 2045 hrs onwards (own room if possible).			
④ a) All toilet requisites to be made ready by 2000 hrs. b) Encourage him to bathe. c) Praise appearance afterwards.			

Fig. 9.1B   Raymond Smith's interim care plan (cont'd).

he and Raymond did not get on well. She therefore allocated it to herself till lunchtime. Progress notes were checked and the care plan modified according to Raymond's progress. She also decided to request that the doctor review Raymond's medication to enable him to sleep at night. The morning itself passed reasonably un-eventfully, and at lunch-time Jane Adams, the nursing auxiliary, was assigned to spend some time with Raymond. His parents arrived shortly afterwards and, after spending some time first with the doctor then with Raymond, Jenny Wright joined them for a discussion on the points she had picked out of their earlier telephone call.

FIRST WEEK

Raymond's presentation gradually deteriorated during the first few days as he became more and more frustrated by his surroundings. His parents stayed for several days and it was apparent that all was not well between father and son. After their visits, his parents would always complain about his behaviour to the staff and they were obviously hurt by his attitude towards them. He was sleeping better by the end of the week and had established some relationship with members of his nursing team. His friends at the university, with one exception, did not visit at all, despite several enquiring phone calls to the ward.

Jenny Wright and her team modified the interim care plan several times to try to cope with the pattern of Raymond's behaviour. They had been able to deal with several immediate problems but still were unsure about the more long-term elements of his presentation. On the fourth day after admission, they started working on the interview, having constructed a nurse's impression. This preparation was carried out on a joint basis with all members of the team discussing their own input to the progress notes. The final nurse's impression was written by Jenny Wright.

Comments

In some cases, the nurse's impression can be constructed at the end of a period of several days, or it can be written out on a daily basis by each individual nurse involved. Where there is considerable written information, due to changing behaviour patterns, involved psychiatric symptoms, or a large amount of information source data, it may be more prudent to précis the total documentation, extracting only the most relevant facts (Fig. 9.2).

NURSE'S INTERVIEW

The interview was carried out by Jenny Wright over a period of three days. The areas to be dis-

cussed were highlighted by all members of the team, including Raymond himself who had become increasingly interested in the activities of his nurses. The areas to be discussed were:

- Why did Raymond feel that he had been brought to hospital?
- What did he expect from the nursing staff whilst he was in hospital?
- Why did he feel that he had difficulty relating to strangers in his environment and why did he become aggressive towards them?
- How did his psychiatric symptoms affect his ability to concentrate and orient?
- What made him feel most comfortable?
- Why did he seem to be more hostile towards males than females?
- What did he hope to do when he left hospital?
- Could he still cope with university life?

Comments

Many of these areas are discussed outside the formal interview and, consequently, very often the comments recorded by the nurse are not those arising from the interview. This does not matter in any way. In truth, the interview is initiated as soon as the nurse meets the patient. What is important is that the nurse does meet the patient and that she gets, and records, as clear a picture as possible of the patient's overt behaviour (Fig. 9.3).

ON-GOING CARE PLAN

From the nursing impression, the nurse's interview and the modification made to the interim care plan, Jenny Wright felt that she had enough information to assess Raymond's situation. She highlighted the following points in conference with her team.

Maladaptive behaviour in Raymond's presentation

Biologically based:

- Four hours sleep only each night.
- Will not eat regular meals.

- Reasonable attention to personal hygiene.
- Little exercise.
- Complains of stomach ache.

Psychosocially based:

- Poor communication with males.
- Interrupted communication with females.
- Indifference towards surroundings.
- Little social contact.
- Afraid of his environment.
- Frightened by his father.
- Confused by his hallucinations.

Biological needs not being satisfied:

- Sleep.
- Eating (food).
- Exercise.
- Freedom from pain (real or imagined).

Psychosocial needs not being satisfied:

- Freedom from fear.
- Communication.
- Orientation/mental awareness.
- Self-expression.

Need priorities

On-going need priorities	*Nursing Diagnosis*
Freedom from fear:	Feels threatened by his environment and those within it.
Sleep:	Sleeps only four hours per day.
Communication:	Becomes abrasive when approached, especially by male staff.
Exercise:	Remains in his room for most of the day.

These findings were then discussed with Raymond who, despite his obvious difficulties with concentration, accepted that they were a fair reflection of his life at the moment. He still felt that he was not abrasive towards people and could not see the need to communicate with them, especially if he did not like them. Jenny Wright decided that it was not a question of

disliking people but more that of simple avoidance.

The remainder of the needs were recorded in the progress notes, and it was decided to place them in the following order of priority:

- Freedom from pain
- Food
- Orientation/mental awareness
- Self-expression.

These needs might well be satisfied before they appeared on the care plan, as they were closely linked with those already being dealt with. The nursing intervention necessary to satisfy the priority needs, would also be appropriate for meeting those temporarily relegated to the progress notes.

Both Jenny Wright and Paul Williams discussed the nursing intervention with Raymond, and this had the effect of making him feel quite important, and he said so. His objectives were also discussed. This meeting was the most successful they had had, but it was marred by a final outburst of verbal abuse from Raymond towards Paul. It appeared to coincide with a discussion on increased mobility and feelings of pain within his stomach. Jenny Wright had already checked with the doctor to see if the medical examination had shown any abnormality with Raymond's abdomen, but there was no evidence to suggest that this was the case. The results of routine investigations had also been negative. The team had decided to relegate the feelings of pain to a lower level of importance because they felt that it could be dealt with by increasing his ability to communicate and his self-confidence, and by reducing his feelings of fear and apprehension. The situation mentioned above seemed to show that their decision was a sound one.

Comments

In the initial stages of care planning, it is important that the patient feels he is involved with what is happening around him. If he is deprived of responsibility and the opportunity of decision-making, it may well have adverse effects on his motivation and commitment to his care programme. One way of maintaining the high level of involvement

Progress Notes

Nursing impression

Full name: _Raymond Smith_ Name preference: _Ray_

Clinical area: _Bowthorpe Villa_ Hospital number: _57032_

Observational period: _1.6.91 – 4.6.91_ Nurse's signature: _SAFbR_

Information source: _Patient, Personal Data, Friends, Parents, Pts. Doctor,_
Nursing Team, Sleep Chart.

Date	
1.6.91	**Patient**: Raymond is a 19 year old university student admitted on 1.6.91 at 1000 hrs. On admission he was relatively quiet, seemed a little disorientated and showed little interest in his situation. He complained of bad feelings in his stomach and refused refreshment. When questioned he became abrasive and refused to answer. He asked about why he was here, what had he done wrong and seemed bitter towards the police, who had escorted him. He seemed to be suffering from auditory hallucinations which interfered with his train of speech. He was dishevelled and unkempt and stated he had not slept for 2 days. He wanted to see a doctor.
	Since admission he has become more disturbed, verbally aggressive towards male members of staff, slept very little, kept away from social contact, prefers the solitude of his own room and has begun to establish a working relationship with his team nurses. His personal hygiene has improved, but he eats very little. He still complains that something is 'eating at my stomach.'
	Personal Tutor: States he has always been rather quiet but appears to have the usual circle of friends. Works reasonably well in his studies.
2.6.91	**Friend**: Mike Williamson. Came from the same part of the country. Not particularly close at university but says Raymond has always been something of a loner, though well liked. Thinks things have been going wrong for him for about 2 or 3 months. Has lost interest in hobbies and social scene. Always complaining of stomach pains, but eats reasonably well.
	Parents: Visited for last 3 days. Seem close but Father/Raymond are always arguing. Mother says he is not like her Raymond, much more 'moody' and 'snappy'. Father says that he thinks his son dislikes university but does not want to admit it.

Fig. 9.2A Raymond Smith's nursing impression.

Progress Notes Continuation

Date	
	Nursing Team / Doctor: Find him difficult to nurse because he is unpredictable. Seems to enjoy writing his thoughts down. Gets on well with female staff. Doctors notes outline auditory hallucinations, thought blocking and depersonalisation.
4.6.91	*Sleep Chart*: Records a maximum of 4 hrs sleep per night.

Fig. 9.2B   Raymond Smith's nursing impression (cont'd).

established during the first few days, is to ensure that the care plan is discussed with him at length and with as many of the team present as possible. This creates the feeling that it is an important event and one which the patient is not only involved in, but is actually the central figure.

The objectives were set at the same time as the nursing intervention was discussed, and Raymond was instrumental in outlining them.

- *Problem 2*. Is able to move freely around the ward area.
- *Problem 3*. Achieves a sleep pattern with a minimum of 6 hours.
- *Problem 6*. Explains how he feels when approached by staff members.
- *Problem 7*. Walks around the hospital grounds in company once each day.

With problem (7) it was decided that Raymond would be accompanied by either a member of the team or, if possible, one of his visitors or even another member of the patient group. When all this information had been transferred to the care plan, review dates set and Raymond made aware of them, the on-going programme was then in progress. Little disturbance had been created in the general pattern Raymond was gradually becoming familiar with. The sister on the ward was briefed as to the general decision of the team and agreed with the basic outline of the plan.

A new care plan was produced as all the initial objectives had either been achieved, or the emphasis upon each problem was different and needed expressing in a more descriptive fashion.

NURSING AUDITS

Jenny Wright examined her own performance on a daily basis. She did this at the handover sessions, and considered such factors as whether or not she had actually carried out the nursing intervention she had allocated herself to give, and her effectiveness in working on the care plan with her team. In Raymond's case she decided that both she and her team had done reasonably well during the initial days of his hospitalisation. There had been few outbursts and his behaviour certainly did not reflect that which he exhibited before he arrived. They had managed to keep the level of medication he received to a minimum by allowing him freedom of expression without criticism and assessing his immediate needs apparently quite accurately. She was concerned about his lack of self-confidence and the decline in his greatest asset, his intellect. She hoped, however, that by allocating priority to the needs as she had done, the combined use of medication and nursing intervention would eliminate the necessity of producing specific care for dealing with this problem.

Nurse's Interview

Full name: _Raymond Smith_   Name preference: _Ray_

Clinical area: _Bowthorpe Villa_   Hospital number: _57032_

Interview date(s): _4.6.91 6.6.91 6.6.91_   Nurse's signature: _(signature)_

Interview

Item ① _Why do you think you are in hospital?_

response
'My stomach is not right'
'I need to get something done about it'
'I don't suppose it is wise to go swimming in the middle of the night'
'All people who do things wrong in society are punished in some way — that's the state'

Item ② _'What do you expect from the nursing staff here?_

response
'Not a lot you can do except get me out and I don't suppose you will'
'Do something about my stomach'
'Talk about my experiences'
'I don't really know'

Item ③ _'Why do you become abrasive towards people in your environment?_

response
'I wasn't aware that I do'
'I don't mean to, but sometimes I get confused.'
'I think people shout at me too much'

Item ④ _'How do your stomach feelings and the confusing feelings_
(his term for his auditory hallucinations) _affect you?'_

response
'I can't eat properly and I certainly can't concentrate'
'I can't read my work or anything'

Item ⑤ _'When are you most comfortable'_

response
'When I am on my own, no that isn't true'
'I prefer talking to someone, no that isn't true either'
'I don't like being out there (the day area, lounge, recreational areas) because everyone there is odd.'
'They make me feel cold — inside'

Fig. 9.3A   Raymond Smith's nurse's interview.

Side two

Item ⑥ 'Why are you more hostile towards males?'

response 'I think it is the other way around'
'I am not hostile to that chap on nights'
'My father is always getting on at me'
'I don't argue with Mike' (Williamson)

Item ⑦ 'What do you hope to do when you leave hospital?'

response 'Go back to University and get my degree'
'Then I will go abroad and live in somewhere quiet'
'I haven't really thought about it'

Item ⑧ 'Can you still cope with University life?'

response 'You know I want to go back to University so really, I
don't understand why we keep talking about it.'
'I am quite capable of doing the work'
'I don't need the people'

General impression of patient during interview(s)

The interview was carried out over a three day period because
it was difficult to keep to the subject. Raymond appears to
be unable to concentrate and may be suffering from thought
disorder, possibly thought blocking. Became quite agitated
at times despite being fully co-operative with the idea of
the interview

Fig. 9.3B Raymond Smith's nurse's interview (cont'd).

The team's performance was reviewed at the weekly ward meetings when all were present. It was generally felt that Paul, the EN, should spend more time with Raymond and the care plan was adjusted accordingly. All said they felt wary of Raymond and put this down to his unpredictability. Members of other teams on the ward said they had little contact with him as he tended to seek out his own nurses. This was encouraging, as it showed he was beginning to trust Jenny's team. The sister remained concerned about Raymond's behaviour towards people who asked him to do things he did not wish to do, and spent some time with the team members discussing their individual approaches. Again, the care plan was modified accordingly.

RAYMOND'S PROGRESS/DISCHARGE

The progress notes written on Raymond were very comprehensive, and the team had made great efforts not to record repetitive information

Patient Care Plan

Patient name: ...Raymond Smith...... Clinical area: ...Bawthorpe Villa.........

Date	Nursing diagnosis	Patient/nursing objectives	Review date
7/6/91	② Feels threatened by his environment and those within it.	② Become able to move around freely within the ward area.	14/6/91
7/6/91	③ Sleeps only 4 hours per day.	③ Achieve a sleep pattern with a minimum of 6 hours sleep.	14/6/91
7/6/91	⑥ Becomes abrasive, especially when approached by male member of staff.	⑥ Explain how he feels when approached by staff member.	21/6/91
7/6/91	⑦ Remains in his room for most of the day.	⑦ Walk around the hospital grounds in the company of his allocated nurse once each day.	14/6/91

Fig. 9.4A Raymond Smith's on-going care plan.

Primary nurse: ...Jenny Wright........... Sheet number: ..2.................

Nursing interventions	Evaluations	Date	Nurse's initials
②a) To be encouraged to sit and talk in different parts of the ward. b) Spend at least 5 mins with him if he approaches you. c) Let him express his own feelings.			
③a) Encourage him to talk in his own room during the late evening. b) Reduce sensory stimuli after 2200 hrs.			
⑥a) Do not interrupt him when he is speaking. b) Continue with experience diary. c) Question his behaviour and get him to try to explain how he feels when abrasive. d) Only allocated nurse to deal with this item. e) Congratulate him when he says how he feels.			
⑦a) Select a time to go for a walk and arrange this with Raymond. b) Get Raymond to choose the route. c) If he wishes to go more often, encourage him.			

Fig. 9.4B Raymond Smith's on-going care plan (cont'd).

and to document only the changes that took place in his presentation. Consequently, problems that were encountered which did not require long-term planning were dealt with using the SOAP note approach. For instance, during Raymond's fourth week in hospital another patient on the ward asked him if he would help him with a crossword puzzle. Raymond accepted but it was soon obvious that he could not concentrate sufficiently to be of any help to the patient. Instead of retiring gracefully, he argued over every clue and every solution until it developed into a slanging match between the two of them. A male nurse spoke to them both and attempted to placate them. The other patient apologised but Raymond stormed off the ward. Since he was now an informal patient this in itself was not a problem, but his frame of mind gave rise to some concern. Paul went after him and eventually they both returned to the ward with Raymond more relaxed but unwilling to mix with the other patients. As this was deemed part of his on-going problem it was not necessary to modify the care plan in any way, but the incident needed to be recorded so that the team could use it in their reviews. Paul recorded the following in the progress notes:

25/6/91   S: Raymond stated that other patients on the ward are testing him and trying to make him seem 'simple minded'. He felt that he had to get away before something bad happened to him.

O: He argued with another patient (male) over a crossword puzzle and stormed off the ward when a male nurse intervened. He became more subdued when I spoke to him in the grounds but on return refused to leave his room.

A: Psychiatric symptoms still appear to affect his ability to concentrate and he felt threatened by the other patient's ability.

P: Will talk to him again about his diary and see if he can explain the situation for himself.

Paul Williams.

The plan was carried out successfully and within a short space of time Raymond was once again back in the recreational area of the ward. In this way the progress notes were felt to be complementary to the care plan and helped in the assessment of Raymond's ability to reach his objectives.

In all, Raymond spent nearly 10 weeks in hospital. Before he was discharged he was visited by the community sister who was going to act as his follow-up support. They agreed on a routine for visiting that would not jeopardise Raymond's standing at the university, and extended his remaining objectives to include the expected problems associated with discharge. His major needs had been met by him while on the ward and he had had the opportunity to examine his own behaviour and approach to other people. His psychiatric symptoms had disappeared by the sixth week in hospital, and the remaining time had been spent looking at his future, his personal objectives and his life plan. On his own admission he was not the person he had been before his period in hospital, but he felt that he could learn from the experience. He was optimistic about his future.

The team reviewed his care after his discharge and his care plans were placed before an audit committee for analysis. It was felt that he had reacted to the change in his life-style, from the shelter of his home to the organised chaos of the university, in a maladaptive fashion. He was not mentally prepared for the change that would take place and the nursing staff had offered him the opportunity to examine his own behaviour and shortcomings and re-design his life-style so that he could cope with it. This was done by setting objectives in the later stages of hospitalisation centring around relaxation and life planning. The audit committee felt that Jenny Wright had organised the care with insight and sensitivity, but felt that she should have spent less time with Raymond herself and given more autonomy to the junior members of the team. The teacher for the learners was satisfied that they had been involved to the extent appropriate to their level of training.

FINAL COMMENTS

This case examines the initial aspects of providing care in a detailed fashion. It highlights some of the problems that psychiatric nurses experience, e.g. patients' unpredictability, threatening behaviour, and lack of immediate knowledge about the reasons for patients' actions. The care plans involved throughout the whole stay in hospital would run to several sheets, but as the patient begins to think more about his discharge he becomes less dependent on others to set his objectives and provide nursing intervention. The general pattern is one of:

- finding out what the problems are
- meeting the needs
- setting out a plan for future satisfaction of the needs
- re-designing the social sequelae that produce the problem in the first instance.

The last area is always a stumbling block if it is approached unrealistically. Re-designing in this context does not mean direct involvement with marriages, unemployment or living accommodation but rather re-designing the patient's response to these situations so that his behaviour is more appropriate. It is important that nurses do not spend too much time dealing with the initial problems leading to admission but look towards the future, isolating areas where the individual can be helped to become more self-sufficient. If he can be helped in such a way that he teaches himself not to react in an inappropriate way to his life-style, he will be better equipped to deal with his life problems. Consequently, the case study does not dwell on the somewhat repetitious care plan review and modification, because the principle remains constant throughout the patient's hospitalisation.

Nurses must not be afraid of looking at the patient, the care plan, the progress notes and the initial interview and saying, 'I cannot find any more areas of need that we can help him with'. At this point discharge must be imminent. Raymond's case was successful because the nurses quickly isolated his main need areas and delivered interventions which did not intrude on his dignity. They established the reasons for his behaviour very quickly, and were able to produce a nursing process which complemented the medical commitment and created an individualistic atmosphere that had both purpose and direction.

SUGGESTED READING

Eccles J 1987 Adventures into individualised care. Senior Nurse 7(4): 12–14

Krebs M-J, Larson K H 1988 Control: a key concept in the management of aggressive behaviour. In: Krebs M-J, Larson K (eds) Applied psychiatric – mental health nursing standards in clinical practice. Wiley Medical, New York, pp. 271–290

Stevenson M 1984 Problems remain: trying to implement the nursing process in an acute area of psychiatry. Nursing Mirror 158:1 Mental Health Forum. V–VII

Ward M F 1988 Psychiatric nursing: current practice. Nursing Standard June 25th: 30–31

10

The nursing process in community psychiatry

INTRODUCTION

When an individual is admitted to a psychiatric hospital it is because he is no longer able to receive appropriate care in the community. It may be because he has become a danger to himself or to others, or it may be that the resources necessary to help maintain his independence are not available. In this context, the hospital offers something unique. It is a resource unit that offers a variety of complex therapies and approaches that would otherwise be denied the client. However, it is also designed to be only a stopgap: psychiatric hospitals, units attached to large general hospitals or wards within the general environment are viewed today less as long-term resting places and more as areas of re-training for return to the community. The nursing process helps provide the link between the two concepts of institutional care and community care, because it identifies the specific problems the client has in coming to terms with his environment: it develops objectives which will enable him to become independent once again and then delivers the interventions to bring about that change. The next step is for the client to return to his own way of life and use the skills he has perfected.

It would be foolish to suggest that, despite this re-training programme, the patient can do this on his own. He stills needs support and guidance and, if necessary, modification of his new objectives. This comes from the community team, and the most important member of this group is the community psychiatric nurse. Barratt (1989) states that many psychiatric nurses in the community have difficulty in separating their role from that of the social worker, but if they adopt the nursing process as their method of care delivery, this role identity crisis can be averted. Social workers are responsible, in the main, for providing services which will enable the individual to pursue a more comfortable way of life. They do provide counselling services, but it is not their job to teach people to help themselves. The nurse, however, using the process, becomes the facilitator of change that enables the individual to seek the satisfaction of his needs through his own skills. The social worker offers the individual support, which will involve a degree of dependence; the nurse offers the individual the opportunity to become independent of her. If the individual is going to achieve some form of recovery, then being dependent upon another person for the relief of suffering is not the answer. The nurse has at her disposal knowledge of the individual's own potential and is, therefore, capable of achieving far more success in the long term. Both nurses and social workers have their roles to play in the provision of community mental health but they should not confuse these roles or eventually the client will suffer.

The hospital, then, provides the crisis cover (although, as will be discussed later, this is not always the case) and the community nurse the long-term back-up and resocialisation agency. This chapter will (1) see how, by using the nursing process, the community nurse can satisfy these requirements and improve the client's ability to perform independently, and (2) consider ways that the nurse may improve on the current scheme.

The chapter has been divided into four main sections:

1. The link between the hospital and the community.
2. Special considerations for the community nurse using the nursing process.
3. Implications for psychiatry.
4. A care study illustrating the use of the process within the community.

THE HOSPITAL/COMMUNITY LINK

As the nursing process is an approach to care delivery used by the vast majority of nurses in psychiatry in the UK, it follows that the clinical and community-based staff should be able to link their work effectively (Pollock 1989). Also, because the process is more than an administrative tool, the transfer from hospital to community, for both the patient and the nurse, will be much easier. Several important aspects of the use of the process are isolated below and examined in the light of the patient's requirements; from this it will be seen that they make the move from the relative confines of the hospital ward to the harsher reality of society a more natural progression.

LIAISON

The community nurse must attend the case meetings before the patient is discharged to discuss the progress made in the problem areas identified by both staff and patient. She must also get to know the patient and discuss with him any problems he is experiencing because of his discharge home. In this way, she initiates her own observation and assessment of the client's need pattern, compares it to that already identified by the ward-based team and decides on any new approaches that can be adopted prior to the date of discharge.

Through her visits, the community nurse can begin to form a rapport with the client which should aid them both in planning any necessary interventions or modifications in the existing care plan. She can begin to develop an understanding of the problems she will have to deal with, and may get the opportunity to meet with relatives and friends who will act as her colleagues while she works with the client in the community. These meetings while still in the relative safety of the hospital ward will give her the time to think clearly about her strategy.

These visits also give the client a chance to meet the person who will act as the hospital representative when he is discharged. They show that she cares about him and that she wishes to listen to his perception of his forthcoming transition from client to member of the general public and all the changes that this entails. As a result, the nurse will have a better understanding of her client and will be better equipped to help him in times of crisis. If he has already had experience of problem-solving techniques whilst hospitalised, he may well look forward to a continuation of this procedure under the guidance of the nurse.

This continuity of care ensures that the client will not be abandoned on discharge to fend for himself, and this may well give him the confidence to face it more positively. Some of the uncertainty has been removed; he has met the nurse; she is not just a person who may or may not come to visit him when he is at home. It is true that much of this can be done without the use of the nursing process, but it is not so effective. If the nurse is to have a clear picture of the client's need pattern, she should spend some time in conversation with him. She must prepare herself for his discharge in much the same way as he himself must, because she cannot afford to make any mistakes. When he is discharged, she must know exactly what she is going to do, when, how often and why. If the process of going home is handled in such a way as to create a massive increase of stress and anxiety for the patient, it will be counterproductive and may well precipitate an early return to hospital. As a result of his experience, the health team are likely to have far more difficulty getting the client home at the second attempt.

CONTINUITY OF CARE

Through the liaison process, the methods adopted by the ward-based nurse can be continued by the community nurse. Continuity is the basis on which the planning process is built. For the client, the prospect of being discharged from hospital, with all the changes that this involves, is a daunting prospect. However, if the care provided by his nurse remains the same, this will give him at least some degree of stability. If the ward staff notify the community nurse several weeks before an anticipated discharge, she has adequate opportunity to familiarise herself with the interventions that have been employed. She may feel that they are inadequate for the task of rehabilitation and she may therefore be involved in restructuring the programme prior to discharge. In this way, the community nurse can ensure that she is capable of meeting the needs of her client with the resources of the community.

EVALUATION OF HOSPITAL INTERVENTION

Because the ward-based nurse has a tendency to view her client's needs in relation to his stay in hospital, it is often difficult for her to design objectives suitable for the client's eventual return to society. If he is to take an active role in society once again, the period of preparation takes place in the final few weeks before discharge is absolutely vital. If the client has been prepared incorrectly, whether due to a lack of nursing insight or of his own involvement, he may well return to hospital within a very short period of time. If the community nurse can become involved in establishing these final objectives, using her special knowledge of the situation that will exist for the client once he has left the confines of the ward, this particular crisis can be averted. She should be included in team discussions and take a leading role in the latter stages of the planning process. The ward-based nurse must be prepared to relinquish control of the care plans, realising that her most effective role is placing the client in the hands of the person now best suited to help him satisfy his needs.

The community nurse should receive a care plan summary from the primary nurse indicating the final stages of the clinic-based programme. Of course, the community nurse should also have a re-admission document that she can use to pass on information about the community care plan for clients who must return to the clinical areas once again. This continuity link is not just good practice but part of clinical reciprocation and the basis of effective communication between the two sets of nurses.

MONITORING THE CHANGING NEED PATTERN

Through her regular visits to the client, the community nurse will be able to establish how the individual's need pattern develops. By using the nursing process, she will be able to assess his ability to achieve the agreed objectives and decide whether or not he is being successful. Because she will not have had the same contact with the client as her ward-based colleagues have had, she will have to devise objectives which are very easy to evaluate. She will also have to make them much easier to achieve as she will not be able to encourage him in the way he has been used to whilst in hospital. She will have to use relatives and friends as her ears and eyes, much as the charge nurse on a ward uses her support staff. She will also have to bear in mind that much of what she is hoping to achieve will be on a support basis and not oriented towards substantial change. Essentially, the community nurse should be instrumental in the individual being able to maintain himself within the community. She is not trying to change his way of life or transform him into a world famous pianist. She must consider him as an autonomous individual trying to take his rightful role in society, and she must use whatever tools she has at her disposal to evaluate his ability to remain as such.

If obvious changes take place, the community nurse is ideally situated to re-design the care she is providing or even, in the most extreme cases, organise a re-admission. It must be remembered that the nurse visiting a client in his own home, at a day centre or at his place of employment, is at a disadvantage when compared to her hospital counterpart. Due to the restrictions imposed by her time schedule, she will have fewer opportunities to carry out comprehensive assessments. Hers is more of a working relationship, and, in most cases, she will deal with only the more obvious problems expressed by the client. She must ensure, therefore, that her criteria for establishing priorities is both efficient and effective. In the transition stage from hospital to home, she will be able to gain professional information to help her from the appropriate staff, but once the client has been discharged she alone will be responsible for organising the implementation of the nursing process. It is, therefore, inevitable that much of the responsibility for ensuring that the correct intervention is being offered, will fall upon the shoulders of the client himself, and the nurse must be prepared to give him as much opportunity to express himself as possible.

In practice, many clients stay on the books of their community team for a considerable length of time in one form or another: for example those who receive depot injections of major phenothiazines, those receiving constant support and counselling and those who simply need to be visited on an occasional basis for a friendly chat and a re-assessment of their present situation. During these visits, the process of teaching and the process of nursing continues in just the same way as before, except that any objectives that are devised are of a long-term nature and should have a very low priority in relation to nursing input. It would be wrong to assume that the nursing process will eventually increase the number of discharges from nursing care responsibility; in fact, the discharge rate is more likely to decrease because the nurse will tend to identify more specific problem areas than she would have using a non-scientific method of evaluation and assessment. What should be reduced, however, is the amount of intervention the nurse is required to give, because the nurse is teaching the client and his relatives to overcome their own problems and meet their own needs rather than doing these tasks for them. This may mean that she has more clients on her caseload but needs to visit them less. Adopting the nursing process makes for a more effective use of the nurse's skills and offers her greater flexibility in the use of her valuable working time. The extra time she needs to spend with her clients before discharge is counterbalanced by the decrease in time she needs to spend with those she is already responsible for in the community.

SPECIAL CONSIDERATIONS FOR COMMUNITY PSYCHIATRIC NURSES

Outlining a system of healthcare delivery which is broadly similar to the approach already adopted is one thing, defining those areas that need to be improved, renovated or completely re-designed to ensure that the system works successfully is another. If the community nurse is to become involved in the nursing process, she will need the same support, guidance and re-education as any other member of the profession adopting on a new methodology. For example, who will provide her with the technical information necessary to educate her in its use? Who will encourage her to be both scientific and creative in her approach? How will she compare her own actions with those of her colleagues? Who will support her and help her develop new ideas? Who will help her audit her actions and monitor her use of time? The answers to these questions and several others considered below are not easy to formulate because different structures operate in different parts of the country and some health authorities have devised their own specific approaches to these and similar difficulties. However, the basic requirements of the community-based psychiatric nurse are outlined below:

- Training and re-education programmes
- Teaching role: patient-oriented
  relatives-oriented
  colleague-oriented
  multi-disciplinary-team-oriented
- In-service education
- Development of new techniques which reflect the nurse's autonomy, e.g. crisis intervention
- Nurse management involvement
- Legal implications of the documentation system surrounding the nursing process
- Research commitment
- Setting up of new projects which centre around nursing process assessments
- Setting up of community nurse referral systems which are not based on psychiatrist or medical officer initiation
- Creating autonomy for community-based psychiatric nurses.

EDUCATION

The training programme for community staff must reflect a patient-oriented approach, but only nurses just beginning their training will benefit from a re-structuring of the curriculum. Those already qualified need a re-education programme because, working in the community as they do, contact with other members of the nursing team is limited and thus the possibility of sharing ideas and techniques is reduced.

However, in many respects, community staff have an advantage over their hospital colleagues when it comes to using the nursing process. This advantage stems from their existing role. The community nurse cannot offer the 24-hour coverage that the patient receives in hospital, instead, many of her visits to him in his home are taken up with teaching him and his family how to deal with the problems that hinder him in his present situation. The nursing process too involves teaching but in a planned and objective way, so that the only new element introduced in the change from one method to another is the care plan (Fielding 1983). In-service education must take into account the existing activities of the nurse and extend them to include care plans and the use to which they are put (Hall 1982).

Making relatives, friends and even workmates an integral part of those plans, and gaining their cooperation and assistance, must form a large part of the teaching curriculum. Other paramedical staff who also act in a supporting role in the community should be made aware of the planned activities of the nurse. Often this can be done by the nurse herself; with the aid of the care plans, she is much better equipped to show just what it is that she and her patients are trying to achieve, how they are intending to go about it and how these support groups can best be utilised to produce the optimum amount of assistance. Probably one of the best ways of constructing the in-service training so that it suits the requirements of the nurse, is to present the nursing process, including documentation etc., to all grades of staff and then allow them to implement the idea. Over the next few months, they make a personal list of the difficulties they encounter and submit them to the teaching staff who produce study days designed specifically to deal with these problems. There should also be a link member or community representative on any nursing process interest group that exists in the base hospital; he or she can put forward the views of the community team and seek advice on possible approaches to dealing with common problems, including educational directives (Altschul 1989). The community team must also find time to meet as a group to discuss their difficulties and share the experience of dealing with them.

DEVELOPMENT OF NURSING ROLE

The nursing process also offers the community nurse the possibility of expanding her role and spreading her expertise. It should be possible, through careful planning of visits and work load, to introduce new techniques of caring for the psychiatric client. All too often, people are admitted to psychiatric hospitals because there is no suitable alternative. The nurse can be that alternative. Crisis intervention, either on a multidisciplinary level or using nursing resources alone, lends itself to the systematic pattern of the nursing process, as the care plans can be left in the individual's home and used as the basis for discussion during subsequent visits. In this way, people can be supported in the community.

THE NURSE MANAGER

The nurse must have the support of her line managers, who must be prepared to set up such schemes as nurse-based clinics, crisis intervention teams, day centres and groups, interest groups, etc. Their management commitment must include active participation in process interest groups, working parties and pilot schemes. They must be able to identify problem areas and have the expertise to offer advice or alternative approaches to solving them (Simmons & Brooker 1986). They cannot afford to become a passive element in the changing pattern of events that will certainly accompany the implementation of the nursing process, otherwise they will lose credibility amongst their own staff. They must be aware of allocation techniques and assessment criteria as well as documentation and administration responsibilities. As a teaching element, they are vital to the on-going education of their nurses. The

opportunity they have to see and speak with every member of the team on a regular basis means that ideas and concepts discovered by individual members can be passed onto others. They are in an ideal position to act as representatives on process interest groups. Consider also the situation where a community nurse goes on holiday or is taken ill, the case load must be shared amongst her colleagues and usually it is the nurse manager who must take responsibility for the increase in work. With care plans in situ, this is a simple task to perform, because all the information necessary to offer the clients their required care is documented in the care plans. Hence, continuity is maintained by the nurse in the clients' homes without the trauma of hospital admission and the added difficulties that this may impose.

Nurse managers must become actively involved in any of the new ideas that their teams elect to use. Like their hospital counterparts, they must 'lead from the front'. If the nurse is to be successful in any initiatives she takes, the manager must provide active support. As a result, managers as well as the other members of the team are able to maintain continuity without too much difficulty.

LEGAL IMPLICATIONS

The nurse must realise that her responsibility to maintain medical confidentiality may be compromised by leaving a confidential document in a client's home where it may be seen by any number of people. However, this is not necessarily a problem because the care plan is designed by nurse and client together, so that the client himself is fully aware of the contents; if he should decide to show it to other people either for discussion or for advice, that is his prerogative. The care plan should not contain medical information and is, therefore, not likely to contravene any ethical code if seen by others. On the contrary, it may often provoke useful criticism from those who care enough to read it.

What is more important to the nurse is the contents of the document. By writing down the activities she intends to pursue, she is committing herself to a course of action and is duty bound to follow it through. If she fails to do so, this will become common knowledge and she may be open to a charge of professional misconduct or even negligence. Both of these have serious implications for the nurse. In a court of law a great deal of importance is placed on documentary evidence and this includes nurses' care plans and progress notes. Should they show that the nurse failed to carry out a prescribed course of care on behalf of the client, it will take a great deal of persuasion to convince the court that the nurse was justified in her failure to do so. This high degree of accountability must be seriously considered when the care plan is initially produced, and the nurse must be sure that it is feasible for her to deliver the care she has designed. Obviously, where there is considerable family or support group involvement, the element of accountability is reduced for the professional, but she still has to monitor the effects of the care and modify the plan where necessary. Failure to do this may result in similar legal consequences.

This raises the question of whether or not the progress notes should also be left in the client's home. They are an integral part of the process documentation and extremely important as a complementary record to the care plans themselves, but it is felt that they should remain with the nurse so that she has access to progress without having to visit each and every home on her round. At case conferences, they can be used as a basis for discussion as they are an account of the client's response to his care plan and, therefore, adequately suited to the task.

RESEARCH

As with hospital-based nurses, it is part of the community nurse's role to become actively involved in scientifically demonstrating that what she is doing is worthwhile and effective. She must consider new ideas with an open mind and, once explored, be prepared critically to evaluate her findings. For too long nurses have relied on anecdotal support for their work; if true professionalism is to be achieved the nurse must become aware of the basic rationale for her actions. The nursing process provides an excellent research tool, both from the point of view of establishing what the effects are on client care and of the nurse's effectiveness in her chosen interventions. Research, of course, becomes a worthless task if it is carried out simply for research's sake, but if small scale projects are designed with a view to increasing the nurse's awareness of her job then it serves an extremely valuable purpose. Some examples of research that the community nurse might initiate from a nursing process standpoint are listed below.

Client oriented

- Client's response to care plan activities.
- Client's attitude towards combined care plan.
- Client's response to his care before and after the introduction of the nursing process.
- Client's involvement in his own care planning.
- Family commitment to care planning and its effects on client progress as a whole.
- Effects on client/nurse communication patterns.
- Client's ability to become independent of the nurse.
- General client progress.

Nurse oriented

- Effects on inter-disciplinary communication.
- Time factors involved with prescribed nursing actions.
- Quality of care provided.
- Time spent with individual clients.
- Size of case loads.
- Personal efficiency in using the nursing process approach to individualised care.
- The production of problem-oriented indexes.

Nursing process oriented

- Whether or not the nurse is using the nursing process.
- Whether or not it affects her attitude towards her care delivery.
- How the nursing process system of client-oriented care might be improved.
- Documentary/administration developments.

Carrying out research for personal use is only valuable to the profession as a whole if the results are shared. Once the community nurse has carried out a small scale research project she must, by virtue of her isolated working conditions, record her findings and distribute them amongst her colleagues. If possible, they should be sent to professional nursing journals for nationwide distribution so that all community staff can benefit from her experiences.

NEW PROJECTS

Research can often be a practical activity, though pure information gathering for analysis at a later date does not always have the same appeal for nurses. Whenever one of the nurses involved in small scale research work considers that she has some worthwhile evidence to support a particular change, it should then be the responsibility of her colleagues to institute small scale pilot schemes to verify her findings. In the community, where much time is spent establishing just what the nurse can offer the patient, the setting up of pilot schemes based on various types of nursing assessments may well improve the effectiveness of the nursing process approach to this job.

NURSE REFERRALS

If the community team can produce assessment tools which suit their role, there is no reason why they cannot increase their responsibility to the primary care team. In the majority of places in the United Kingdom, most clients are seen by the community psychiatric nurse as referrals from a psychiatrist. Usually, these referrals occur because an individual is being discharged from a psychiatric hospital. However, there is no reason why 'non-in-patients' should not benefit from the services as often the nurse has the skills and techniques which can make a hospital admission unnecessary. Either a social worker or the client's family doctor should refer directly to a community-based psychiatric nurse who, equipped with her own variation of the nursing

process assessment tool, can utilise the resources at her disposal to effect meaningful nursing intervention as an alternative to uprooting the client from his own environment.

IMPLICATIONS FOR PSYCHIATRY

With any introduction of new ideas and concepts into an existing structure, there are bound to be considerable repercussions. For the psychiatric nurse who implements the nursing process within a community setting, these repercussions may be very far reaching. Questions will have to be asked about staffing levels, finance, individual roles and multi-disciplinary activities. By using such a system, the emphasis of the whole of nursing care delivery is altered. Developing her skills to a more advanced and scientific level may mean that the nurse becomes frustrated with a traditional system that does not move with her. The result of such frustration may be that she leaves nursing altogether or becomes bitter and insular in her work. The resultant lack of communication in such a situation will prove counterproductive for the client. It is, therefore, worthwhile considering how the psychiatric nursing services may be affected by the use of the process, and how they may develop to ensure that they benefit from its obvious advantages.

We have already seen that for the community nurse the use of the process means an increase in her responsibilities. The nursing interventions she may decide to use may well be considered by other disciplines to lie within their own sphere of activity. This should not deter the nurse. If she feels that she has the capability to provide a particular type of care and it is in the best interests of the client that she do so, then she should act accordingly. One of the main reasons why psychiatric nurses have lost much of their traditional therapeutic work to other professional groups, is that they have consistently failed to demonstrate control over their work and develop it to enable the more spontaneous delivery that only nurses can provide. By showing competence in those neglected areas, the nurse can regain much of the credibility that may have been lost over the years, and present nursing as a scientific, creative and autonomous discipline. If the nurse develops into a therapist, there is no reason why she should not be able to prescribe the care either in a complementary fashion, where other groups of health professionals are involved, or totally independently, where she is the only representative. Mental health clinics, administered and staffed by qualified psychiatric nurses using nursing process techniques, may be one direction in which the community staff see themselves progressing. Active involvement in therapeutic groups, day centres and mobile hospitals may be another. Existing merely as a support group for discharged patients is not a way of using the community nurse's skills to their full potential.

COMMUNICATION

It is perhaps in the field of communication that the nursing process should have most impact on the community nurse. With the aid of the care plans, she has a tool with which to demonstrate her actions to other members of the primary care team. She must increase her communication with the other groups and avoid the danger of working in isolation (Johns 1990). Often, where members of more than one discipline are involved with the same client, they can be providing similar support without the knowledge of the other's activities. This is confusing for the client who ends up as piggy-in-the-middle with little chance of receiving benefit from either of his would-be helpers. It is therefore important that support personnel are aware of the nurse's interventions with the client so that they can produce programmes complementary to hers. Community occupational therapists, voluntary workers, etc all have their roles to play in the patient's development, but they must be coordinated by the nurse and included in her system of referrals. The need for such specialist help will be ascertained by the nurse doing her assessment of the patient's problems and included in his care plan as an appropriate resource or substitute for nursing intervention.

This increase in communication should have further benefits. The nurse working in the field of mental health must also pay attention to those people diagnosed as being physically ill. For community psychiatric nurses, this may mean two things. Firstly, they may be asked by general nursing staff to assess potential clients in general medical/surgical wards prior to discharge and ascertain whether or not any actions may be necessary on their return home. Secondly, they may be asked to provide psychiatric nursing intervention for those clients once they have been discharged. The use of effective assessment criteria and a systematic method of delivery for the required care are invaluable for these tasks.

CASE STUDY

The following case study is designed to show the individualised way in which a CPN applies the theory of the nursing process within a community setting. As will be seen, the unique aspects of social setting, limited contact time and the amount of shared responsibility within the client/CPN relationship demand a professional methodology which other disciplines would find difficult to replicate. This methodology is closely allied to the original philosophy of nursing process, thus making the delivery of effective clinical support a more attainable goal.

CLIENT BACKGROUND

Gary Mendham lives at 21 Hall Road with his wife and two young children. He is 33 years old and works for a local baker. Over the last 8 years he has been admitted to the psychiatric unit of the local district general hospital on three separate occasions following serious disruptions in his ability to achieve a safe, practical and satisfying lifestyle.

It seems that whenever Gary is confronted with difficult problems in his life, such as moving house, changing job, children being off school through illness, money shortages, marital disharmony, etc., he goes through a series of changes in his behaviour which ultimately leave him unable to cope with even the simplest of personal tasks. Prior to his last admission he was extremely rude to his employer and threatened to smash up his bakery if he did not get his own way. He expressed feelings of extreme agitation, which resulted in a breakdown of all his personal relationships; he imagined that unspecified others were plotting against him, which made him a source of ridicule, thus fuelling his beliefs; he found it impossible to hold meaningful conversations with anyone, leaving him misunderstood and feeling even more insecure; he became easily discouraged with minor projects if they did not go as he intended; he lost interest with his family and friends and eventually he withdrew from all forms of social contact reacting aggressively to those who tried to get involved with him. As a result of this he was extremely unhappy, both with himself and his predicament, finding it virtually impossible to satisfy even the most basic of his biopsychosocial needs. His children became frightened of him because he behaved so strangely towards them and this had a dramatic effect upon his wife who had all but left him.

The home situation became intolerable and eventually Gary was re-admitted following the intervention of the CPN. It later transpired that much of Gary's behaviour was a response to the increasing pressures placed upon him by an ever more demanding young family.

HOSPITALISATION AND DISCHARGE

During his stay in hospital Gary had managed to come to terms with most of his negative feelings, though he still retained those of distrust and isolation. He had become far more capable of identifying and dealing with his own need requirements, almost to the point of full personal competence. This was partly as a result of his active involvement in the planning and development of his own care programme under the guidance and direction of his primary nurse. The result of this was that he was far more aware of the changes that had occurred in his behaviour and, perhaps more importantly, why they had taken place. He had managed to recognise aspects of his life which generated high levels of stress, and considered ways in which this affected his body and his thinking and how to identify these changes when they began to occur. Finally, he had examined a series of alternative life strategies designed to help him cope in a more positive and satisfying way with both the pressures when they occurred and the effects that they had on him. The CPN had been involved only in the later stages of Gary's stay in hospital, when the 'action plan', designed to test the strategies, had been evaluated. Gary had made numerous trips out into the community and the CPN had monitored his progress.

The CPN visited Gary on two occasions prior to his discharge so that they could re-establish their working relationship and work out the basis of their activities together once he was home again.

On the day of discharge, the CPN drove Gary home and stayed for a short while to confirm the contents of their contract. Gary's wife had been at home but said or did very little that could have been regarded as a welcome home for her husband.

Comments

It can be seen that the arrangement that exists between the client and the CPN differs appreciably from that experienced within an in-patient facility. Firstly, the CPN already knows a great deal about his client and has had the opportunity to see him functioning within a variety of settings. More significantly, he has seen the client within his own environment so that the intervention he offers is geared more towards the provision of positive help and support; this is in contrast to the situation in hospital, where the client tends to rehearse things more often than actually use them. Secondly, nearly all of the initial observational material has been gathered prior to the client becoming part of the CPN's active caseload. Thus, the evaluation of such material can be carried out in a far more informal fashion, with each visit or contact point being regarded as a possible opportunity for change.

Interim care plan evaluation

The CPN, Tony, left Gary's home and drove for a couple of miles in the direction of his next visit. He pulled into a side road and, having parked his car, reflected on his session with Gary. He needed to construct a picture combining both what he already knew and what he had just witnessed. Several sources of information were at his disposal:

1. Gary himself
2. Gary's wife
3. the in-patient documentation
4. Gary's primary nurse
5. his own community records and progress notes made during his visits to Gary both before and during the last admission.

The information from these sources had already been carefully considered, primarily in the construction of the interim care plan (Fig. 10.1), but Tony needed to establish whether the most recent impression he had of Gary – that of a reasonably competent individual – corresponded with that he had just displayed on leaving hospital. After all, he and Gary had agreed upon a series of actions and if these were no longer relevant they would need to be up-dated. As the interim plan itself was open to question it was necessary to carry out a review straight away, and for several reasons:

1. The interim care plan was constructed whilst Gary was in hospital and therefore did not

necessarily represent his true aspirations and desires now that he was home once again.

2.   The objectives around which the plan was produced were relevant whilst Gary was in hospital, as they represented his perception of his needs at that time. These may have changed even in the short time since his discharge.

3.   Gary's expectations of both himself and those around him will have been influenced by the sense of well-being generated by the institutional system. Again, once at home this sense of well-being may have deserted him.

4.   The level of stress that Gary experiences is likely to have risen since leaving the hospital, and all his previous difficulties have resulted as a consequence of such an event.

5.   Tony can make only an educated guess as to what Gary will do once he has settled in at home; there is therefore a degree of built-in obsolescence in the original planning; it is almost 'disposable'.

Nursing diagnosis

The nursing diagnosis had been a simple statement relating to Gary's general behaviour prior to discharge, and not one reflecting his overall problem:

'Is concerned about how he will behave once he arrives home.'

Tony was reasonably happy about Gary's performance both on leaving the hospital and when eventually they arrived at his house. He felt that Gary had coped well with the changes inherent in being discharged from a large institution, and he had an air of determination that suggested he was equipped to deal with his wife's apparent indifference to his homecoming. The nursing diagnosis was, however, still relevant, because no one, including Gary himself, was sure how the next few days would progress. In fact, it was the behaviour of Gary's wife that troubled Tony more than anything else.

It was as important for Tony to examine the environment in which the expressed diagnosis was likely to manifest itself as it was to examine Gary's response to it. Whilst in hospital, Gary had been in a position to exercise a certain amount of control over what happened to him, but now, back in his own home, he would have to consider the demands of others as well as his own. In effect there were far more variables at work within Gary's own home than had ever existed whilst in hospital, and the greatest of these was his wife. It was she, rather than he, that might determine the success or failure of Gary's endeavours. However, at this point Tony felt that he did not have enough information about the marital relationship to be able to decide upon a future course of action, and made a note to investigate during the next visit.

Objectives

Satisfied with the accuracy of the nursing diagnosis, Tony next considered the objectives he and Gary had agreed on.

1.   To identify warning signals that might suggest that stress is becoming intolerable.
2.   In the event of No. 1 occurring, to use one of the selected pre-arranged strategies to cope with the experience of stress.
3.   To discuss areas of difficulty that appear to cause greater stress than others with my CPN.

Tony was also satisfied with the content of the objectives, especially as Gary had not actually achieved any of them at this stage. Their suitability would be evaluated at the next meeting, when Gary would review his own progress.

Comments

Several factors are worth noting at this stage. Firstly, there are three separate objectives for the one problem. This might appear to contradict the principle that each problem should have only a single identified objective, but on careful scrutiny it can be seen that each of these objectives leads to the next to form a continuum or string. Such a series enables contingencies to be catered for without the need to construct complicated sets of possible or potential problems. It allows for variations in the client's own performance and encourages relative successes, as opposed to absolute success or failure.

Secondly, it can be seen that all of the objectives are of an expressive or experiential nature. It would be unsuitable for such a series to include a behavioural objective, for such an objective requires an absolute response. Gary's objectives are not prescriptive in this way, but allow him the opportunity to achieve them as best he can and not necessarily in a set fashion.

Thirdly, the objectives in this string work in a cyclical way with a form of evaluation built into them, the third in the series being written in the form of a discussion. By doing so they create an on-going situation, constantly giving rise to further attempts at achieving objectives (1) and (2). When being formally evaluated it is unlikely that they will need to be altered, because they can accommodate any changes in the intervention programme.

Patient Care Plan

Patient name: _Gary Mendham_   Clinical area: _Community_

Date	Nursing diagnosis	Patient/nursing objectives	Review date
11/2/91	(8) Is concerned about how he will behave once he arrives home.	(8) a) Identify warning signals that might suggest that stress is becoming intolerable. b) In the event of Nº1 occurring to use one of the selected pre-arranged strategies to cope with the experience of stress. c) Will discuss areas of difficulty that appear to cause greater stress than others-with my CPN.	16/2/91

Fig. 10.1A   Gary Mendham's interim community care plan.

Finally, by constructing such a string of objectives the CPN enables the client to perform at his own level whilst still having some control over the sequence of events. It is unlikely that such a sequence would be used in the same way within an in-patient facility, because here the response to the intervention programme could be monitored more closely by the care team. In the community, however, the nurse has to give far more responsibility to the client and by producing such a string the element of risk or failure can be reduced.

Data review

Next, Tony needed to review the observational material he had obtained whilst with Gary in his home. As things stood, the current nursing diagnosis and it's subsequent actions all related to the problem of leaving hospital and coming to terms with being at home once again. This diagnosis would need to be updated at some point, and Tony had to begin to construct a profile, of both Gary and his environment, that could form the basis of this. His review of the data, including Gary's home situation, was carried out using the same biopsychosocial formula as is used by Tony's ward-based colleagues.

Physiological

1. Gary was reasonably fit, strong and healthy.
2. The home was well maintained, tidy and comfortable.
3. Gary's wife seemed physically well.
4. No sign of the children but the wife had said they were well.
5. There were no observable reasons why Gary could not physically cope with home life.

Primary nurse: _Tony Smith (CPN)_		Sheet number: _3_	
Nursing interventions	**Evaluations**	**Date**	**Nurse's initials**
⑧a) To use one of the agreed stress coping strategies already used. b) To attempt relaxation once signs of 'over stress' occur. c) To try to find his own way around stressful situations.			

Fig. 10.1B   Gary Mendham's interim community care plan (cont'd).

6. House was close to shops, children's school, pub, work place and the homes of some of Gary's friends.
7. Gary did not have a car, but then he did not need transportation at present and, if necessary, there was a bus-stop close to the house.
8. Gary was reasonably active.
9. Gary's wife made no physical contact with him when he arrived home.

Of these observations Tony decided that (1)–(8) were positive, with only (9) being seen as possibly negative.

Psychological

1. Gary was a little concerned at what people might think of his having been in a psychiatric hospital. He had often said that after his previous discharges this had been the most difficult thing to come to terms with. Tony listed this under psychological, as opposed to sociological, observations because very often the problem did not rest with other people. They were in fact often very tolerant and understanding. The difficulty rested more with Gary who firmly believed that others would feel strangely towards him; it was therefore something that he himself had to come to terms with.
2. Gary was on a 'high' as far as personal achievement was concerned. He felt he would be able to cope with his life using the new strategies.
3. Was looking forward to going back to work.
4. There was still some doubt about Gary's ability to recognise his own stress responses.

Of these observations, Tony regarded (2) and (3) as positive, and (1) and (4) as negative, although Gary was aware of (1) so that this too might constitute a positive factor.

Sociological

1. Gary had chatted merrily about all sorts of things whilst in the car but had tended to be more subdued on arriving home.
2. Felt that being admitted to hospital had been a positive experience for him.
3. Was looking forward to being re-united with his children.
4. Seemed reasonably at ease.
5. Did not intend to contact his friends or workmates just yet.
6. Had hinted that he felt one or two people pointed him out whilst in the street as being someone who had been inside a psychiatric hospital.
7. Did not appear to be aware of the coldness with which his wife had greeted him, instead he justified her position by saying that he had been away for the last three months and she was bound to feel a little uncomfortable.

Of these observations, Tony regarded (1)–(4) as positive, with (6) and (7) being a little disturbing though not necessarily negative. Observation (5) seemed natural in the circumstances, but in conjunction with (6) might pose a problem in the future.

Nursing intervention

Tony made note of all this data and had several options open to him. (1) He could adjust the care plan to accommodate some of the negative points he had observed, but this would be unfair to Gary who would know nothing of the alterations. (2) He could ignore the negative issues and carry on with the existing plan, but this would also be unfair to Gary because it would mean that he never had the opportunity to discuss Tony's observations with him. (3) Tony could leave the care plan as it stood, making sure that it was evaluated against the backdrop of these observations at the next visit. Tony chose the third of the options because this would give Gary the time and space to organise himself, whilst also generating the feeling that Tony trusted him to carry out his part of the care contract, i.e. the work involved with the care objectives. Tony also felt that he would be making extra, and perhaps unnecessary, work for himself to simply change the care plan every time things did not seem to be going according to plan. Gary needed to be given the opportunity to show what he could do for himself, and altering things before he had the chance to get settled would only confuse and dishearten him.

However, this outwardly passive form of intervention needed to be discussed with the other members of the care group at the next team meeting so that everyone was aware of what was happening and to ensure that objectives were not compromised

by well-meaning, but ill-advised, intercession on the part of others. Tony also needed to get more information about the family unit from their social worker to see if there were any clues concerning Gary's rejection by his wife.

Comment

Having agreed a course of action with his client, the CPN had to keep his end of the bargain and allow the client the opportunity to do the same. Had the CPN's concern for the marital relationship caused him to return earlier than agreed, the client might have seen this as a lack of trust in his abilities, or simply had his equilibrium disrupted by a change in plan over which he had little or no say. Removing the element of decision-sharing would have shifted the power balance in favour of the CPN and left the client feeling that he was being manipulated in some way by the nurse. Generating the sensation of 'nurse knows best' within a community nursing setting will only produce helplessness in the client, or, worse, resentment and anger which is not necessarily always expressed towards the nurse responsible. The CPN also needed to give his client the opportunity to assert himself within his own household once again, and to find out if the wife would become more supportive of her husband.

It would seem that, in many ways, the CPN has to take certain calculated clinical risks within the therapeutic structure of the client/nurse relationship that are not outwardly present within an in-patient facility. The nursing process allows the CPN the scope to document, structure and justify the nature of those decisions at the moment they are made, thus providing the rationale for actions as well as the time scale for carrying them out.

FIRST FOLLOW-UP VISIT

After 5 days Tony visited Gary at his home once again as originally agreed. He was surprised to find that his wife had gone out shortly before he arrived and was not due back until later that day. This was not necessarily significant, but as he had hoped to gauge the warmth of her response towards Gary it was a little disappointing.

The first few minutes of the visit were spent discussing general items of interest, and gradually Tony brought the conversation around to the care plan. It was Tony's belief that the care plan should form the basis of all his home visits to all his clients. It gave him a substantial reason for visiting and provided shape and dimension for his interviews. He had noticed that his clients quickly got used to the approach and seemed to be relaxed and comfortable with it. They had often said to him that they felt it made their care seem important and he was convinced that the continuity it gave his visits contributed to the good relationships he had established with those clients. Gary was no exception to this rule and was quite happy to continue in this way. Their first task was to evaluate the effectiveness of the existing plan of action. As always, they began with the objectives.

Evaluation of the care plan

Objective 1

All of the objectives had been negotiated prior to Gary's discharge from hospital, but it soon became evident that something was wrong. Despite the intensive work that had been carried out, Gary had apparently not been as capable of recognising his stress thresholds as had been imagined. He admitted to several outbursts during the last few days which appeared to have been precipitated by such things as difficulties with his children, his role in the management of household affairs, financial matters and feelings about his next door neighbours. More significantly, he did not appear to be able to identify these precipitators, and it was left to Tony to talk the incidents through with him so that they made sense.

Objective 2

As a consequence of this failure to achieve the first objective the second one had not been successfully achieved either. Again, Gary was not aware of this; he kept repeating that he understood what he was supposed to do, yet had to be reminded of what it was.

Objective 3

This was the main discussion point between them. Tony realised that Gary would not be able to tackle the first two objectives until he had begun to appreciate his interactions with the things going on around him. This objective, essentially expressive in nature, was therefore achieved, although it would remain on the care plan to be used again at the next visit. Only the method of achieving it would alter, being dependent solely upon Gary's responses.

They talked for an hour and finally agreed to cut the amount of objectives to number three only. There was no definable outcome for this objective, only that Gary would try to achieve it in his own way. The objective statement was altered so that it reflected the actual needs of the moment:

'I will think about what has made me angry the next time I feel that way'.

Client action

As there was nothing that Tony could do in this situation to contribute to the outcome of the objective, no intervention was recorded. Instead, the actions that Gary would need to carry out were discussed and documented. These included:

1. Trying to involve Gary's wife in the discussions.
2. Asking her if she would be present at the next visit.
3. Making notes of things that seemed important.
4. Trying to find things that cropped up more than once.
5. Sitting somewhere quiet after the angry incidents.
6. Trying to sort out if there was anything in particular that happened to Gary when he got angry.

This last entry was the beginnings of an attempt by Tony to help Gary recognise, if not the precipitors, at least the behaviour he used. If stress factor analysis failed, then it might be possible to get Gary to identify the behaviour associated with loss of control and counteract it before it got out of hand.

All this information was placed on the on-going care plan.

Nursing diagnosis

They agreed that it was not necessary to change the original statement because Gary was still trying to come to terms with the problems associated with returning home.

Tony was still unsure about the wife's involvement but decided not to tackle the subject head-on with Gary in case he compromised his relationship with him. He made a copy of the care plan (Fig. 10.2) for Gary to keep and refer to at his leisure, and simply mentioned in passing that he hoped he would be able to say 'hello' to Gary's wife the next time he called. Having agreed upon a time and date for the next visit, Tony left.

Progress notes

Once again the progress notes were written whilst parked in a lay-by. Tony documented all those elements of the interview which gave some indication of Gary's strengths and weaknesses. He did not document here specific information about why the

Patient Care Plan

Patient name: _Gary Mendham_   Clinical area: _Community_

Date	Nursing diagnosis	Patient/nursing objectives	Review date
11/2/91	(8) Is concerned about how he will behave once he arrives home 16/2/91	(8) a) Identify warning signals that might suggest that stress is becoming intolerable. b) in the event of N°1 occurring to use one of the selected pre-arranged strategies to cope with the experience of stress c) Will discuss areas of diffi-culty that appear to cause greater stress than others - with my CPN.	16/2/91
16/2/91	(9) Gary became agitated without realising that it was happening.	(9) "I will think about what has made me angry the next time I get that way."	21/2/91

Fig. 10.2A   Gary Mendham's on-going community care plan.

Primary nurse: Tony Smith (C.P.N)	Sheet number: 3		
Nursing interventions	Evaluations	Date	Nurse's initials
(8) a) To use one of the agreed stress coping strategies already used. b) To attempt relaxation once signs of 'over-stress' occur. c) To try to find his own way around stressful situations. 16/2/91	Evaluated in Gary's home – CPN/client. Objective (8) a) Not achieved. Objective (8) b) Not achieved. Objective (8) c) Should be rewarded and used to develop the on-going care plan.	16/2/91	TS
(9) a) Sit down quietly after incident and try to work out what has happened. b) If I have any real ideas about the event I will write them down on the paper provided. c) I will discuss these feelings with my wife. d) I will talk to Tony about these ideas at his next visit.			

Fig. 10.2B Gary Mendham's on-going community care plan (cont'd).

care plan had been changed, because this had already been done on the care plan evaluation section. To duplicate this information would have been time-consuming and superfluous. The progress notes provide only the background information for this work. However, Gary did identify several priorities from the information he had gathered, one being a reminder for himself to make sure that Gary was aware that he was to make progress in his own time and not be ruled by what he thought Tony might require of him.

Comment

It can be seen that the ways in which the CPN carries out his assessment and executive activities are far more informal than those of his ward-based colleague, following the same infrastructure yet not always in the same order. It is essential that the nursing process is carried out at the client's own pace and in a way that best suits his personal requirements. The object is to make the process fit the client, not vice-versa. It is perhaps true to say that a greater degree of freedom exists within the client/CPN relationship than anywhere else within the psychiatric discipline, simply because the CPN is not in a position to monitor, guide, support and intervene within the executive elements of the care plan. In this particular case, the CPN has contact with the client for perhaps only one hour per week and therefore it is the client who must dictate the style, nature and intensity of the care. As a consequence, real equality within the relationship can be achieved, for as the realities of trying to lead a satisfactory life influence the client so the care becomes interwoven with the complexities of actual problem solving. Fewer objectives are set, more parameters need to be identified within the care structure, and significantly more trust is given the client. In short, by virtue of their need to give their clients more responsibility, CPNs are potentially closer to using the nursing process as it was originally conceived than are many other members of the profession.

SECOND FOLLOW-UP VISIT

At the next visit, Tony was pleased to see that Gary's wife had decided to stay and meet with him. He was able to establish that she had some serious reservations about her husband's behaviour, and during the conversation Gary became agitated and moody. Tony was in a position to discuss this response in relation both to Gary's feelings and the contents of his care plan.

Gary's wife agreed that she had a significant part to play in the outcome of any objective that Gary set

himself, and it was concluded that she would begin to take an active part in both the evaluations of the plan and, to a lesser degree, some of its construction. Although there was obviously some doubt as to just how effective she could be, her attitude seemed positive and Tony was able to leave the house feeling that at least Gary had an ally with whom he could explore the possibilities of a more realistic care programme.

Final comments

As with all care plans, any person who is actually involved in the care programme may be included on the care plan. Within the community, this may include friends, neighbours, relatives or even pets, as long as they have something to contribute. Care planning has the added bonus of providing these support personnel with both a sense of purpose and a medium through which it can be expressed. The CPN might never be in a position actually to confront the family relationship problems which may be at the heart of a client's behaviour, but at least he can stimulate a working dialogue, using the nursing process, which might give all parties concerned greater insight into each other's needs. In Gary's case he was able, through a long, and sometimes painful individually-constructed programme, using a sequential approach to self-awareness, to resume a more rewarding and meaningful lifestyle. Without the nursing process it is unlikely that the programme could have been sustained.

SUMMARY/CONCLUSION

By introducing the nursing process into the general format of the community psychiatric nurse's daily activities, the whole concept of psychiatric nursing can be altered. Being able to demonstrate to other members of the multidisciplinary team just what it is that she is doing with her clients enables the nurse to increase her role and become a more active member of that team. To do this, however, the community staff must first develop their own special methods of assessment, for it is in this area that the hospital and community adaptations of the process differ. In hospital, the nurse has a longer period of time in which to gather her data, and much greater client contact with which to evaluate her findings. The community nurse has no such luxury. She can increase her contact time by visiting the patient in hospital prior to discharge, making use of data already gathered and adding to it, using her own more specific assessment.

Using the process in the community is not just about the relationship that exists between client and nurse, it is about utilising resources and facilities that are outside the domain of the health worker. It is about developing the role of the nurse to include that of coordinator linking the client with the most effective method of teaching him to gain or regain independence. It is about increased communication with other members of the health care team and establishing the nurse as the most important person within it. Moreover, it is about bringing psychiatric nursing to all those who need it, whether they be psychiatric clients, general clients or simply the man in the street who feels he can no longer cope with what is going on around him. With the aid of the nursing process, this is possible.

REFERENCES

Altschul A 1989 One or many? Community Psychiatric Nursing Journal 9(6): 14–18
Barratt E 1989 Community psychiatric nurses: their self perceived roles. Journal of Advanced Nursing 14: 42–48
Burgess A W 1981 Psychiatric nursing in the hospital and the community, 3rd edn. Prentice-Hall, New Jersey
Fielding J 1983 Teaching is part of nursing. Journal of District Nursing 1(8): 28 : 32–33
Hall V 1982 The community mental health nurse: a new professional role. Journal of Advanced Nursing 7 : 3–10
Johns C 1990 Autonomy for primary nurses: the need to both facilitate and limit autonomy in practice. Journal of Advanced Nursing 15: 886–894
Pollock L C 1989 Community psychiatric nursing: myth and reality. R.C.N. research series. Scutari Press, Harrow
Simmons S, Brooker C 1986 Community psychiatric nursing: a sociological perspective. Heinemann, Oxford

SUGGESTED READING

Buchan T, Smith R 1989 Nursing process in community psychiatric nursing. Australian Journal of Advanced Nursing 6(3): 5–11
Gray D E 1986 Community and institutional roles: evaluation by Australian psychiatric nurses. Community Mental Health Journal 22: 147–159
Stoul B A 1990 Community support systems for persons with long-term mental illness: a conceptional framework. Psychosocial Rehabilitation Journal 12(3): 9–26
Ward M F, Bishop R 1986 Learning to care in community psychiatric nursing. Hodder & Stoughton, Sevenoaks

11

The nursing process in continuing care psychiatry

INTRODUCTION

Traditionally, the person entering a psychiatric hospital is likely to stay for a longer period of time than his medical/surgical counterpart. However, due to advances in therapeutic techniques and changes in attitudes that have occurred during the last 20 years, the tendency towards protracted periods of hospitalisation has been reversed. The current approach is to either keep people out in the community rather than admit them, or get those admitted back to their homes as soon as possible. The long-stay population has gradually been falling for quite some time, and a steady stream of these patients return to the community every year. The problems that face patients and their rehabilitation teams are enormous and these are exacerbated by the serious shortage of suitable placement areas within the community environment. For a person who has been used to institutional life for anything up to 10–15 years the relearning of social behaviour appropriate to our modern society is a long and arduous process.

Each step of the rehabilitation procedure must be carefully monitored. Recently, much of this rehabilitation has come to be carried out by other disciplines working within psychiatry – occupational therapists, psychologists, etc. The nurse, however, is still the crucial person around whom the team works.

CASE STUDY

This case study looks at a nurse-centred rehabilitation team working on a hostel ward. Unlike the case study in Chapter 9, only a few staff are involved, and their approach to the use of the nursing process is therefore slightly different. The case will be discussed from the point of view of the ward sister, who has a staff of four qualified psychiatric nurses, and a member of the night staff. The hostel, Wilton House, is in the grounds of a traditional psychiatric hospital, but is managed by both patients and staff as a separate unit. There are 12 patients of whom six attend outside employment. The case study will look at a newly transferred patient and the nurses' approach to his rehabilitation programme. He has already undergone 12 months rehabilitation activity prior to transfer.

PATIENT BACKGROUND DATA

Lional Fredrick Grove was 47 years old and had received almost continuous in-patient care for the last 11 years. He was a reasonably alert, cheerful man who had managed to maintain an element of independence throughout his time in hospital. He was medically listed as being schizophrenic but this did little to describe the man.

When he was transferred to Wilton House he brought with him several suitcases of personal items including a collection of match box tops which he proudly displayed in his room. Neat and tidy in his appearance, well spoken and quite spontaneous, it seemed difficult to imagine that he had lived an institutional existence for so long. The team on the ward, led by Sister Jane Moore, showed him around the hostel, then to his room and suggested he get unpacked. Whilst he did so they reviewed the information they had been given about him from his previous ward.

Fred, as he preferred to be called, had lived with his sister most of his life, but when she was killed in a road traffic accident in 1974 he became very withdrawn and sad. He had no other living relatives and eventually his social decline was such that he left his bungalow very little. He lost his job and it became evident that he had been very dependent on his sister to look after him. In 1975, he was admitted to hospital severely disturbed, being hallucinated and deluded. His presentation was essentially that of a very suspicious man.

Despite being discharged, he needed to be re-admitted on three more separate occasions until, in 1978, he was transferred to a modern long-stay ward and had remained there ever since. His stay in that area followed the usual pattern of events, in that he gradually settled into a routine from which he seldom strayed. His symptomatology was such that he remained reasonably effective if left to his own devices but became quite irritable and disturbed if confronted or asked to change. His symptoms and his surroundings combined to produce a situation from which it was almost impossible for him to deviate. In 1991, the senior staff on his ward decided that Fred was capable of far more than he was doing and embarked on a programme of rehabilitation preparation for him. This culminated in him working in the stores department of the hospital three days a week and being transferred to the hostel. His transfer notes pointed to the fact that he was very set in his ways and that this recovery pattern had been achieved only very slowly and by gaining his complete cooperation for every step taken. The main purpose for his being in the hostel was to provide him with the confidence to live outside the hospital and to enlarge upon his work pattern.

RECENT OBJECTIVES

Jane Moore had already met with Fred before his transfer and they had discussed, in the company of his charge nurse, his most recent objectives:

- Produce a list of things he would like to do when he is discharged. (Expressive)
- Visit the city centre to do some shopping in the company of a nurse. (Behavioural)

Both these objectives had been achieved, and with comparative ease. The list gave a very clear indication of Fred's expectations:

- Find a job working in either stores or distribution delivery.
- Have a bungalow of his own with the money he has in his bank account.
- Keep a dog as a pet.
- Move away from the hospital, but not too far.
- Go to the cinema regularly.
- Teach himself to cook.
- Buy a bicycle.
- Get some peace and quiet and find privacy.
- Increase his collection of match-boxes.
- Do what he wants to do whenever he wants to do it.

On his shopping expedition Fred had purchased several match-boxes and razor blades and both he and the nurse had gone to a cinema in the afternoon. It was obvious to the team that much of what Fred wanted for himself was obtainable, but that a lot would depend on his ability to come to terms with the pressures and responsibilities of living on his own in the community. His chances of employment were not good but at least he had a realistic view of what he might be able to do. His sister's bungalow had been left to him in her will, but following hospitalisation had been sold under the orders of the Court of Protection and the money placed in trust for him. Unfortunately, the money had devalued considerably against the rising cost of house prices and he would not be able to buy new accommodation outright. He would need either a short-term mortgage or rented rooms.

Most of the other items on the list were based on his desire for independence and would not necessarily be influenced by either employment or accommodation. Most of them were accessible to him whilst he was in hospital. By examining what he had already achieved, which was considerable, and considering both job reasons for coming to the hostel and those of the nursing staff who had recommended his transfer, it was possible for Jane and her staff to outline the assessment programme.

- Examine how he responds to unusual or unknown situations; look for increases in psychiatric symptomatology.

- Measure his personal effectiveness in a set group of social circumstances.
- Review his work potential with the chief store-keeper in the hospital stores.
- Evaluate his self-sufficiency.
- Evaluate his socialisation pattern.
- Assess his ability to make decisions.
- Assess how he feels about himself in relation to change.

Comments

Very often, on transfer to a ward, much of the data to be discussed will already have been collected and the assessment programme takes the place of the usual observation section. Much is already known about the patient and the team have to establish at what level of rehabilitation he is functioning and what the potential for improvement is. The transfer system can work in two different ways:

1. The patient is transferred, interviewed and the programme is devised.
2. The patient is interviewed in his own ward, the programme is produced and then he is transferred.

Both systems have their advantages and disadvantages, but option (2) does appear to produce a more systematic approach to continuous care and reduces the possibility of transferring a patient before he is ready. Once the programme has been devised, the patient is informed that he will be assessed over the next few days, and various assessment scenarios are set up by the staff to provide the various types of information they need for the assessment. At the end of an agreed period of time, all the data is evaluated and the care plan is produced with the aid of the patient himself.

DATA COLLECTION

Fred was allowed to explore the hostel and told that nothing much would be happening for the first few days whilst he acquainted himself with his new surroundings. He was also told that he would be assessed over the next week and that he should continue to go to work at the stores and carry on his usual social and personal activities. The few rules of the hostel were explained to him, and he appeared to be surprised at the relative amount of responsibility he was allowed. Of Jane's team, all qualified psychiatric nurses, it was decided that only two – Steven Byrnes and Jenny Bishop – would be involved in setting up the assessment programme. Jane herself would act as the coordinator for the team and the data collector. The whole team would carry out the evaluation and care planning at the weekly ward conference the following week. Fred was asked to discuss each day the events that had taken place, his feelings towards them and his attitude towards how he had performed.

Fred was assessed in the following situations:

- His response to his fellow patients, his role on the ward, his behaviour to female patients: he had lived on a single sex ward for all his long stay and it was necessary to see how he coped with sharing his life with females once again.
- The night staff, Rick Little, looked at his social pattern during the evening, his ability to organise his own life routines and activities of daily living.
- He was given a set of jobs to carry out which included his commitment to the work rota of the hostel.
- He was asked to deliver messages and visit, for various purposes, other parts of the hospital that were otherwise unfamiliar to him.
- He was accompanied into the city for an afternoon and allowed to organise the trip for his own purposes.
- He was taken to the job centre and the job hunting system was explained to him.
- His work in the stores was discussed with the chief storekeeper and he was asked to increase Fred's responsibilities so that he had more than usual to contend with.

Comments

The immense amount of information gathering required by a rehabilitation team to ensure that they have a good baseline to work from accounts

for a considerable amount of their time. Unlike the situation on a conventional ward, they do not have a large patient population to contend with, and the majority of their patients are either at work or attending some occupational area during the course of the day. Meal-times, personal financing and social activities are usually run by the patients themselves with the staff playing a merely supervisory role. This means that they are much less restricted than their ward counterparts in the amount of time they can spend in the assessment of the patients' abilities. They also have the added bonus of the patients being more active, thus providing a greater amount of assessment material. The nursing process, therefore, is based far more on observation and evaluation than it is in most other areas. Much of the information gathered may be used by other members of the team, but inevitably the actual decisions about the rehabilitation care plan rest with the nurses. Team conferences are easier to organise, and one day a week they meet to discuss, review and debate the issues surrounding a patient's progress.

In Fred's case, therefore, the observation section of his progress will be carried out by three of the staff, plus the sister, and will be discussed by the whole team. He will be invited to the meeting so that he can discuss the team's ideas, and at that point, when the care has been decided upon by all concerned, one member of the team will become responsible for his on-going care plan.

That person will report back to the rest of the team and seek their guidance and advice in difficult areas. The sister will coordinate the whole programme. Fred will be encouraged to examine his own performance with more objectivity than has been expected of him in the past.

TEAM FINDINGS

At the team conference one week later, Fred's case was scheduled to be discussed first. Consequently, Fred did not go to work that morning. The team made a note that he informed the stores the day before that this would be so. The profile of Fred was drawn up by Jane Moore from the information she received from her three staff, including night staff (Fig. 11.1). The patient interview would be the responses Fred gave at the conference to the profile (Fig. 11.2).

The actual interview was carried out by Jane Moore, though at times Fred did discuss matters with other members of the team. She invited him to air his opinions and, although he was not too forthcoming, he did show that he was quite an intelligent man who could respond well to a stimulating environment. Jane was somewhat provocative towards him because she was not sure whether the shyness he presented was due to lack of personal confidence, or because he felt threatened by those around him. She concluded, after he failed to respond to her, that he lacked personal confidence as his original referral suggested. When asked what he hoped to achieve whilst on the hostel ward he seemed mystified at first, and Jane explained that the objective system he had been used to on his ward was in action there also. He responded quite freely after that.

In his company the team discussed the areas that they felt he needed to work on and asked Fred what he thought. Jane collected all the various suggestions, and it was obvious that most people felt the same way about the direction Fred's care should take. Needs not being satisfied were:

- Physical exercise
- Change in environment
- Affiliation
- Self-expression
- Self-confidence
- Self-identity.

Fred agreed with these and stated that he had never been a great mixer but would like to be able to meet people without feeling uncomfortable. They asked him which of these needs did he feel were a priority. He selected:

- Affiliation
- Self-confidence/self-expression
- Change in environment.

Strangely enough, the work pattern was never even considered as it appeared that Fred could cope with an increase in this area. However, Jane asked Fred if he would include this on his list, and this was agreed.

- Occupation.

The team then converted these needs into specific nursing diagnoses:

- Fails to mix with people on a purely social level.
- Will not initiate conversation.
- Spends too much time in the confines of the hospital and, in particular, his own room.
- Is only working a shortened three-day week.

Next, they set the objectives for these areas. They asked Fred what he thought he would like to achieve first. Not all his answers were realistic but after discussion he agreed on the following as his long-term objectives:

- To be able to talk freely in company without having to leave the room or hide in a corner.
- To initiate conversation with both males and females.
- To spend at least two nights a week out socialising.
- To work a full five-day week.

His short-term objectives were again discussed with him and once again he was responsible for outlining the steps he would ultimately take. Jane Moore helped him to modify them where she thought they were too difficult.

- Will not go to his room till 2130 hours. (Behavioural)
- Will discuss with the nurse how he feels when approached by others during the day. (Expressive)
- Will produce a list of the everyday activities he would like to participate in. (Expressive)
- Will attend work three days/week and occupational therapy departments two days/week. (Behavioural)

At this point, Fred left the meeting and the team had to decide what care they would use to help him achieve his initial objectives. Jane asked for suggestions from the team and it was decided that all those involved in his rehabilitation should

Progress Notes

Nursing impression

Full name: _Lional Frederick Grove_   Name preference: _Fred_

Clinical area: _'Hilltops'_   Hospital number: _39071_

Observational period: _9.3.91 — 16.3.91_   Nurse's signature: _AStJ&R_

Information source: _Patient/Chief Storekeeper/Staff Nurses Steven Byrnes, Jenny Bishop — Night Staff Rick Little, Occupational Therapy Staff._

Date	
9.3.91	**Patient:** Since arriving on the 9.3.91 Fred has remained rather quiet and solitary. There has been no obvious evidence to suggest a flare up of his symptoms and he seems to be quite at ease. His personal hygiene is excellent, his room kept clean and tidy. He seems willing to tackle any task given to him but lacks self confidence when faced by people with whom he is unfamiliar. This manifests itself by him becoming very quiet and a little restless, excusing himself as soon as possible and disappearing either to his room or some other sanctuary

Chief Storekeeper: Has increased Fred's work load and he has responded to the challenge enthusiastically.

S/N Steven Byrnes: Observed Fred mixing very little but getting on well with the female patients. Seems a little threatened by males. Has carried out ward tasks diligently and appears able to grasp the essentials of a situation quickly. Has made excursions to other parts of the hospital on an errand basis with little difficulty though will not linger once his job is done.

S/N Jenny Bishop: Did well in the city. No real problems though he was obviously unfamiliar with the geography of the place. Functioned well in the job centre and understood the difficulty of job hunting.

S/N Rick Little: Sleeps well, without medication. Always tidies his room up before retiring. Enjoys the T.V., plays cribbage, and quite well. Attends to activities of daily living well. Baths each night. No complaints of constipation etc. |
| 16.3.91 | **O.T. Staff:** Is absolutely overjoyed at being transferred to the hostel ward. He is proud of his progress so far and eagerly anticipates his discharge. Seems a little worried about finding a job, especially since he visited the job centre. Takes all his meals in the rehabilitation flat with fellow patients and 2 days a week helps in the preparation, cooking etc. Is rather shy in large groups and does not mix very well, even with people he has known a long while. |

Fig. 11.1 Fred Grove's nursing impression.

Nurse's Interview

Full name: _Lional Frederick Grove_   Name preference: _Fred_

Clinical area: _Hilltops_   Hospital number: _39071_

Interview date(s): _16.3.91_   Nurse's signature: _A.Thp_

Interview

Item ① _Shyness in company of others_

response
'I don't like strangers very much'
'I don't know what to say to people. Sometimes I feel tongue-tied and the only way to make sure I don't make a fool of myself is to keep quiet.'
'I think I could overcome this, but I have always been a shy person.'

Item ② _Relationship with members of the opposite sex_

response
'I like ladies of course'
'They remind me of my sister'
'I don't feel so shy in their company and usually they make me feel like a real person, you know — man and wife sort of thing — like it should be'

Item ③ _Areas of work you most like to do._

response
'I don't mind what sort of work I do but I do enjoy being in the stores and would like a job in a place like it'
'Working with other people would not really bother me if I had a job to do.'

Item ④ _What do you hope to achieve by being here in the hostel?_

response
'I want to get well enough to be able to leave the hospital'
'I want a job and a real life'
'I would like to be made stronger as a person so that people didn't make me feel shy.'
'I want the staff to tell me all the things I do wrong, so that I can correct them and leave with good prospects.'

General impression of patient during interview(s)

This interview took place at the weekly conference and Fred functioned extremely well in it despite being in the company of six other people. Spoke very softly, but with determination. Is obviously trying hard to do his best and overcome his shyness if that is what it is.

Fig. 11.2 Fred Grove's rehabilitation nurse's interview.

be represented on the plan. They checked with the store-keeper and the senior occupational therapist, gaining their cooperation and promising to send copies of the care plan for them to examine. Eventually, when Jane had received proposals from all present, she selected those which she considered to be most suitable.

Comments

As the team leader in this situation, it is the Sister's job to identify all possible approaches to dealing with the problems faced by the patient. She listens to all the various ideas, sifting and sorting them until eventually she isolates a combination that seems suitable. Although after the care plan is completed she will hand over responsibility for it to one of her staff, the initial job is hers; later she will act as an advisor to the allocated nurse. Her initial involvement thus enables her to offer greater assistance to the team in the future. It is not uncommon for care plans, once devised, to be shown to other non-paramedical members of the hospital rehabilitation team, in this case the store-keeper. If such a person is actively involved in a patient's care, it is essential that he is made aware of what the nurses and the patient expect of him. There is no reason why he should not be shown the care plan by the patient himself.

CARE PLAN

The care plan was constructed at the conference, allocated to Jenny Bishop, then discussed afterwards with Fred himself (Fig. 11.3).

Comments

If a patient is transferred from another ward which has been using the nursing process, then the code number for each of the new problems must run in sequence with those already used. In this case, the four new problems isolated are given the numbers 21–24 (Fig. 11.3). In some cases, where patients do not do well in the rehabilitation areas and need to be transferred back to their original ward, this system will reduce any confusion that might exist over problem identification.

For areas such as rehabilitation and long stay, it is not uncommon to find data relating to other areas. Where a patient's nursing programme is linked with that of the occupational therapy department or a work area, then it is important that this fact be identified by the allocated nurse. In this way, communication between the groups involved can be coordinated and the fragmentation of care avoided.

CARE DELIVERY

After the nursing intentions had been fully explained to Fred, and Jenny Bishop had outlined their relationship as allocated nurse/patient, the programme was put into effect. Each week, Fred's case was reviewed at the weekly conference, as the staff always tried to evaluate the programme on either a one- or two-week basis. Jenny Bishop always presented the information to the group and they then agreed, both amongst themselves and later with Fred, on what the next stages should be. The Sister acted as Jenny's back-up on her days off, which meant that she was actively involved with Fred's programme throughout his stay in hospital. Staff other than nursing staff were also involved in the care plan. The senior occupational therapist became involved in Fred's case and the two disciplines linked resources in relation to his social skills training and his personal assertiveness. They agreed on the same objectives and, although there was still some nursing input for the programme, it was largely taken over by the occupational therapy group. The work programme gradually increased until Fred was attending work for four days a week with limited responsibility in the dispatch area. With the aid of the nursing staff around the hospital, his progress in the area of communication was maintained. The other patients on the ward also became an important element in his programme, and one even participated to the extent of being included in the care plan. Jane Moore always worked on the principle that her job was to use all the resources at her disposal in an attempt to reduce Fred's problems. It was thus acceptable to put friends, relatives, staff from other disciplines and even patients on to the care plan.

Fred's progress in the hostel was extremely good. His ward had been using the process for the last 2 years and, consequently, they had prepared him well for his final rehabilitation. He took far more responsibility for setting the objectives of his own care and managed to achieve them all without too much difficulty. After $3\frac{1}{2}$ months he was offered a job by a local firm whom the ward had contacted. His job there would be to act as deputy dispatcher, a role which he had already proved he could handle. It was decided that he should accept the job while remaining as a patient at the hospital, sleeping in the hostel and taking his meals there. When his care plan was constructed to complement this change in the pattern of his life, it was decided that he should be asked what help he thought he might need. His answers formed the basis of the care delivered in connection with those areas still outstanding.

EVALUATION OF LONG-TERM OBJECTIVES

The team initially set target dates for Fred to achieve his long-term objectives and recorded them in his progress notes. It was soon realised that the time span available was not appropriate and they decided to review his progress now that he had reached a critical point in his programme.

Objective 1

To be able to talk freely in company without having to leave the room or hide in a corner.

Evaluation

This had been partially achieved. He was able to maintain conversations with people and, once over his initial shyness, did not try to avoid socialisation. Problem 21 still remained, however and it was felt that by placing him in a work location his ability to communicate with people would be severely tested.

Conclusion

Objective not achieved. To allow a further three-month period before reviving it again.

Objective 2

To initiate conversation with both males and females.

Evaluation

This had been a relatively successful area. He was quite capable of creating an introduction for himself, and had demonstrated this quite early in his stay at the hostel. He was still a little reticent where new people were concerned but the team felt that this was quite acceptable.

Conclusion

Objective achieved. To be considered once again in one month's time, following a period in employment.

Objective 3

To spend at least two nights a week socialising.

Evaluation

Fred had produced a list of items that he wanted to become involved in and had soon become actively engaged in pursuing his own ideas. He had managed to persuade other patients to participate, and although at first he had stayed close to the hostel he now spent sometimes three or four nights at various clubs or social events.

Conclusion

Objective achieved.

Objective 4

To work a full five-day week.

Evaluation

Fred had worked four days a week in the stores and attended groups and classes at the rehabilitation centre of the occupational therapy department. Strictly speaking, this was not five

Patient Care Plan

Patient name: ...Fred Grove...........   Clinical area: ...Hilltops...............

Date	Nursing diagnosis	Patient/nursing objectives	Review date
16/3/91	㉑ Fails to mix with people on a purely social level.	㉑ Will not go to his own room until 21 30 hrs.	30/3/91
16/3/91	㉒ Will not initiate conversation.	㉒ Will discuss with nurse how he feels when others approach him during the day.	30/3/91
16/3/91	㉓ Spends too much time in the confines of the hospital, and in particular his own room.	㉓ To produce a list of evening activities he would like to participate in.	23/3/91
16/3/91	㉔ Is only working a shortened 3 day week.	㉔ To attend work 3 days a week, and OT 2 days a week.	30/3/91

Fig. 11.3A Fred Grove's care plan.

Primary nurse: ____Jane Moore____   Sheet number: __14__

Nursing interventions	Evaluations	Date	Nurse's initials
(21) a) Initiate a personal assertiveness programme - ST/N Bishop. b) Attend social skills group × 3/7. c) Night staff to involve him in all evening social events. d) To discuss, daily, his progress with allocated nurse/key worker.			
(22) a) See No.21 for assertiveness training. b) Speak to him at least once per ½24. Assess response. c) Set aside discussion period after evening meal.			
(23) a) Night staff to prepare list with him. b) Relate items on the list to activities taking place - try to get him interested in something that is happening.			
(24) a) OT staff to monitor effects of OT attendance upon him. b) Chief storekeeper to monitor at work. c) Each dept. to increase responsibility and workload. d) OT dept. to continue existing rehab. programme and liaise with allocated nurse.			

Fig. 11.3B   Fred Grove's care plan (cont'd).

days' employment, but the group felt that it qualified for an achieved rating. Fred's occupational therapist, who had been Fred's link member on the team reported that he had worked extremely hard at social skills, personal assertiveness, and home skills.

Conclusion

Objective achieved. For review in one month's time to assess his ability to work five days in the same area for an outside employer.

General conclusion

The team also agreed to add to this list of long-term objectives because Fred's progress had caused a change in his needs pattern. They considered his future on the ward, his alternatives to hospital and his eventual rehabilitation. It was decided:

- To maintain him on the ward for a period of three months and then start to look for alternative accommodation for him should he progress as steadily as he had done.
- Gradually to reduce the nursing input so that eventually he was maintaining himself totally independently of the team. This would create a better atmosphere for the transition to independence outside the hospital.
- To continue the evaluation process and involve him as much as possible in the structure of his care/assessment.
- To consider his needs in the area of work:
  – transport
  – accommodation
  – finance.
- To introduce him to the Social Services Department and develop a relationship between himself and a social worker.
- To contact the community psychiatric nurse and begin to plan a discharge programme.

With these areas in mind, the long-term objectives agreed for Fred were as follows:

- He should take control of his own care programme and its evaluation under the guidance of his allocated nurse. (Behavioural and expressive)
- He should construct a life plan which highlighted those areas in his discharge that would need to be achieved. (Expressive and behavioural)

These were discussed with Fred and he began to work towards them by setting himself some more short-term objectives.

FINAL COMMENTS

The nursing process in a totally rehabilitative setting is an extremely useful tool. It shows how well a patient is responding to the challenge of his possible discharge and gives both patient and staff an indication of the direction in which the care should go. Preparing a person for a dramatic change in his lifestyle cannot afford to be a haphazard task. It must be done through careful and systematic assessment and evaluation.

Most hostels devise their own assessment criteria based on the resources and facilities available to them. The nursing process becomes not only the method by which the care is constructed but also the philosophy behind its own delivery. The patient has to take responsibility for his own decisions and actions, and the process can be adapted so that eventually he has complete control over his life. Because the level of dependence is greatly reduced in such working areas, the nurse has far more time to spend analysing the effects of her interventions. The approach adopted in the care study is probably the easiest to use in these areas. It means that each nursing practitioner is responsible for her own case load and responsible to the person in charge of the ward. They, in turn coordinate the patient's care and chair the meetings which jointly decide on the individual's scheme. At all times, the other departments involved in the care process must be kept aware of what is happening. Patient problems that are being dealt with by the paramedical groups must be written onto the care plan, as they form an integral part of the nursing programme.

SUGGESTED READING

Armitage P 1989 Primary nursing in long term psychiatric care. Senior Nurse 9(9): 22–24

Davidhizar R, Cosgray R 1990 The use of Orem's model in psychiatric rehabilitation assessment. Rehabilitation Nursing 15(1): 39–41

Norman I, Parker F 1990 Psychiatric patients views of their lives before and after moving to a hostel: a qualitative study. Journal of Advanced Nursing 15: 1036–1044

12

The nursing process in the care of the elderly mentally ill

INTRODUCTION

Whereas the number of classic long-stay residential psychiatric patients is on the decline in the majority of hospitals, that of elderly mentally ill patients appears to be growing. This is due to several factors, both social and medical. Despite the fact that probably as few as 10% of the elderly ever suffer from mental illness during the final stages of their life, there are people with medical diagnoses of Alzheimer's disease, chronic brain failure and organic brain syndrome etc, represented on nearly all of the psychiatric wards. Nurses on acute admission areas may often find that a large proportion of their time is spent with such patients whilst they are being assessed medically, and areas specially designated for the elderly mentally ill are steadily increasing.

Nursing the elderly has always been regarded as a very special job because of the nature of the patient's presentation and their apparent lack of recovery, though acute elderly areas, and assessment units have perhaps had some influence on this. In psychiatry, where these problems are exacerbated by the added factor of psychiatric symptoms, the challenge to the nurse's ability is even greater. When dealing with the common problems of memory loss for recent events, inability to say where you are, who others are and what time of day it is, and general suspicion, it is not difficult to see why many nurses have a pessimistic attitude towards their role. The actual nursing care involved is quite straightforward in many respects, but nurses who perceive their job as a maintenance one will soon develop stereotyped approaches to their patients which deny them any possibility of receiving individual attention. Like everyone else, the elderly have a set of needs which must be met, but their ability to communicate their requirements is impaired by their conditions. They must be nursed in a structured environment which they can relate to, but the nurse should aim for continuity rather than strict routine. The nurse should also aim for an increase in the patient's adaptability to his illness, as opposed to becoming resigned to steady decline and deterioration. If the care is to be stimulating to the patient it must also be so to the nurse, otherwise its quality will suffer. The nursing process offers a framework for action to the nurse involved in this type of work. It creates a meaningful working environment for the nurse and a purposeful and therapeutic one for the patient. Even during the later stages of a patient's illness, where the deterioration is quite marked, the nurse can still provide systematically designed care. During the final stages the nurse is able to offer the patient dignity and respect, whilst still catering for changes in needs. The case study below examines such a situation.

CASE STUDY

The patient involved has been in hospital for a considerable period of time and has reached a point in her illness where deterioration is the only change that takes place in her presentation. The case study will be viewed through the activities of a third-year student nurse currently carrying out the final stage of her training with elderly mentally ill patients. She is a member of one of the two primary nursing teams that work on the ward. The study also takes into consideration some aspects of allocation and time management, and there is some input from the nurse education centre.

DAY ONE

Joy Miller was a third-year student nurse starting her first day on the final stage of her rostered clinical experience with elderly mentally ill patients. As with all ward changes she felt a little apprehensive, but more recently things had become more stressful for her because she was now a senior student. Ward staff expected more of her and in those first few days on a new ward it was always difficult to readjust and assert oneself.

The ward sister welcomed Joy to the ward and said she would speak to her later. She was assigned to Nursing Team A and placed under the supervision of Staff Nurse Keen, primary nurse for the team. She was given a brief tour around the ward and then handed four care plans. These, she was told, were the care plans for a group of patients in a four-bedded cubicle for which Team A were responsible. These were to be her patients for the morning shift.

Joy checked the names on the care plans with those on the patient's beds and quickly ascertained who they all were. Next, she read through the problems and nursing diagnoses that had been made for each one, their specific objectives and the nursing interventions that were required to produce the behaviour outlined by the objectives. She quickly assessed from the plans that she would be able to cope quite easily with three of the patients but would need some assistance with the fourth, a Mrs Emily Graham. The team had a care assistant, an associate nurse who would provide help with Emily.

Joy decided that she would carry out the nursing care required for her first three patients before asking for assistance with Emily. In this way, she could get the feel of the ward and create an initial relationship between herself and her small group. All went well except that Joy was unable to leave Emily until last because she became quite agitated and had been incontinent of urine. Eventually, with the help of the auxiliary, all the special areas of care were attended to, her group had their breakfasts and the morning started in earnest. Staff Nurse Keen gave her a brief run down on the team's responsibilities which amounted to 10 patients. On most shifts there was a primary nurse, an EN and a learner with either one or two care assistants. This meant that each nurse was usually responsible for between four and six patients during the shift, with support from either the care assistants, or, if possible, another member of the team. The primary nurse did not always allocate patients to herself but often acted as a support, particularly for the learners. This meant that she could offer supervision at most times. Unfortunately, on Joy's first morning two nurses had failed to arrive on time and she had to assume responsibility for patient care without the usual supervision.

The two discussed the care plans, the system of allocation and the ward facilities and resources. Joy decided that she had been incorrect in her approach and priority-setting for the care she had to give. Emily should have been dealt with first as the others could probably have managed with very little help from her. However, she decided that this was not entirely her fault as the care plan did not outline Emily's presentation very well. She asked the staff nurse who was responsible for care plan modification and was told that it was carried out by team consultation, with the primary nurse having the final say. Whilst on the ward, learners were made to keep a diary of the care offered to selected patients and they were also given the responsibility of the care plans and any other documentation for those patients. It was suggested that as Joy did not necessarily agree with the care plan for Emily she might like to accept her as her project patient. Joy agreed. She planned her next days accordingly. It was decided that she would:

- Acquaint herself with the team's patients, the care plans and progress notes.
- Become involved with all of the facilities available on the ward for specialist nursing.
- Research through Emily's existing documentation for her background information.
- Modify her care plans accordingly after consultation with the primary nurse.

Joy spent the remainder of the shift carrying out the existing care outlined on the care plan, making a note of the review dates. She also had the opportunity to examine the care plans for the rest of the team's patients.

Comments

It is always difficult to step into an existing nursing set-up and function effectively. The nursing process is able to provide the nurse with up-to-the-minute information about a patient's special needs and what the nurse can do to meet them. It cannot establish the link that is necessary for the patient and nurse to form a relationship, but it can create an atmosphere of confidence and continuity. Unfortunately, there are two problems that may arise.

1. If the care has been written without consultation with other staff it may reflect only one individual's approach and personality. Consequently, when used by someone else it is inappropriate.
2. If the patient's need pattern is not carefully monitored, the care delivered does not actually meet these needs.

The incoming nurse is always at a disadvantage because she must rely on the care plan being correct. If she finds that despite following the care plan she fails to help the patient effectively, she begins to lose a little of her confidence in it. She must establish what, if any thing, is wrong with it, and if she is at fault for the way she has interpreted it. The care plan is vital on a ward such as this. Without the care plan each patient would be got out of bed and made to follow the nurse's interpretation of the routine in spite of their own requirements. Only at a later date, when the nurse was more familiar with the patient, would the style of care alter. That may suit the nurse, but not the patients, who may have to endure several such staff changes each month. The nurse must help the patient to follow the routine events on each ward in his own individual way. By following the care plan the nurse is offered some insight into how this might be done. Certainly, no modification of the plan should be carried out by the incoming nurse until she has had adequate opportunity to get to know the patients concerned.

DAY TWO

Joy spent much of her non-contact time on this shift researching Emily's background and clinical/nursing history. Emily had been in hospital for nearly a year-and-a-half which meant that there was far too much data for Joy to be able to read the whole history of her case. She decided to get a picture of Emily on admission and one of her at the present time, and then draw a comparison between the two to establish the amount of deterioration that had taken place. She studied the various admission documents, including the admission sheet, nursing impression and nurse's interview. The following facts were established:

- Emily was 81 years old, a widow of eight years with one daughter who lived in Canada. She had lived alone for many years and had seemed to cope well until she set fire to the kitchen. The fire was easily controlled by neighbours but Emily became very tearful and distressed. It was apparent by what she said that she was quite disturbed, and careful inspection of her house revealed that she was not particularly safe left on her own.

- On admission she was quiet, distressed and withdrawn. She suffered from recent memory impairment, disorientation and the occasional verbal outburst. She had difficulty walking without support and was incontinent of both urine and faeces on the first night. She refused to eat, and her personal hygiene was poor.

- She was visited by a representative of her local Woman's Institute who had maintained this link until the present day. She had no other visitors. Her daughter wrote to the sister on the ward, but not to Emily, who recently had denied all knowledge of a daughter.

- During her hospitalisation she had initially made some improvement in her ability to meet her physical needs, but she always remained apart from the other patients and became quite angry if they interrupted her thoughts. She had no awareness of her surroundings or her situation. Her memory was still poor though she was able to find her way around the well signposted ward. She was never discharged back to her home because it was felt that without constant supervision she had become a liability to herself and possibly even to others.

- Her property was put in the control of the Court of Protection and her home was sold.

- Her nurse's interview showed that she had never really come to terms with her admission, and the nursing impression highlighted the problems she had interacting with others.

- Her progress notes made specific reference to her talking about her husband as if he were in the next room. She never referred to him as being dead.

- No one seemed to know what hobbies she had pursued and, as she had never been employed, the staff had never been able to refer to her job.

- She enjoyed listening to music, talking to the ward canary and being pushed in a wheelchair around the grounds. She appeared to do little else and spent much of her time asleep.

- She was often incontinent of urine first thing in the morning, needed to be supported wherever she went, could only read the ward signposts with difficulty, never mixed with fellow patients and was quite feeble.

This information gave Joy an insight into the type of person Emily was; it did not give her any warning of her verbal outbursts. As the shift was finishing and Joy had decided on her strategy for the following day, she approached Emily to say goodnight. For several minutes Emily shouted at her, spat at her and even tried to grab her. In the review of the care plans this problem had been highlighted, but it had not been apparent for some time. Joy decided that her next step would be to plot a path through the problems that had been identified to see if any improvement could be made on the present nursing diagnosis.

Comments

Very often when a group of nurses are responsible for a patient's care for a prolonged period of time they develop methods of handling that patient that are never documented fully. Sometimes, they do not even realise that this has taken place. The patterns of interaction that occur between two people usually work in a ritualistic fashion. Various approaches to the other person are tried until the most effective approach is discovered. From then on, that approach is the one which is adopted because it is rewarded by a reciprocal response from the other person. Such behavioural trial-and-error is an innate human characteristic and only the most aware are ever able to analyse what has taken place.

Within the framework of the nursing process this type of subjectivity can pose problems. If the nurses involved do not try to find out why their behaviour is either successful or unsuccessful, their experiences cannot be shared by their colleagues. Consequently, when a new nurse arrives on the ward they must go through the whole routine once again, and, as seen in the situation above, this can be traumatic for the patient as well as the nurse. If the rationale for successful behavioural approaches is fully documented then the new nurse is able to modify her own activities from the onset, thus avoiding disruption of the patient's psychological status quo. If, however, the situation is not outlined on paper, the new nurse has two alternatives open to her. Firstly, she seeks advice from the original members of staff and tries to identify the behavioural approaches that they have adopted to cope with the situation. Secondly, if this is not sufficient she must piece together the information that she can find in the existing documentation and compare it with her own observations. She will need to analyse the situation carefully to find common areas, and once she feels that she has an answer she must record it. If necessary, she may need to place this on the care plan as an on-going problem with appropriate nursing intervention, so that others who follow do not have the same difficulty.

DAY THREE

Problem analysis

The first thing Joy did the following day was to ask her other team members what they did to avoid such dramatic confrontations with Emily. They said that she had been like that for quite some time in the past, but had not had such an outburst for at least three months. They did not know why it took place and could offer no particular approach that would successfully counteract

it. When it had occurred they simply stayed with her until it subsided. They could not recognise a definite pattern of events which triggered it off.

Although they had not realised it, the team had already provided Joy with some useful information. Next, she checked through the care plans to find the last time that this behaviour had appeared as a nursing diagnosis, and what problems were identified with it. Having done this, she then checked to see if the same problems occurred together at any time during the period of hospitalisation. Finally, she cross-checked the progress notes at appropriate dates to establish what the staff had recorded. This included observations and rationale for the care given. She discovered that:

- Aggressive outbursts had been part of Emily's original presentation.
- They had become less marked after a few weeks.
- They had reappeared on the care plan eight times since admission.
- They often occurred when changes took place on the ward, including team changes and new staff.
- A nursing diagnosis of 'becomes verbally aggressive on approach' was usually accompanied by one of 'will not mix with other patients'.
- On three occasions there had been urinary tract infections at the same period of time.
- She was usually nursed by one single nurse during these outbursts.
- She was allowed to vent her feelings without interruption.
- They usually subsided after two or three outbursts.
- They were not recorded as an on-going problem.

This information allowed Joy to formulate a picture of this particular problem. She realised that her plan of action must begin with urinalysis, but she needed to outline a nursing diagnosis which would highlight the problem in the future and enable new nursing staff to deal more effectively with it. She reported her findings to Staff Nurse Keen who suggested that Joy postpone devising her plan till her clinical teacher had visited the ward.

Nurse teacher involvement

Joy outlined the situation she had encountered to the nurse teacher responsible for supervising her clinical activities, and they decided to work on the problem as part of their ward teaching programme. Before carrying out any further assessment, the two worked together with the patients allocated to Joy, and during a lull in the workload the information available was discussed. They compared this information and their knowledge of Emily's present condition with the care plan (Fig. 12.1).

Joy already knew quite a lot about Emily and was able to give details to the teacher.

● Problem 3. This had always been one of Emily's greatest difficulties but it had changed in its presentation over the period of her hospitalisation. Initially, she had been abusive towards others as well as actively avoiding them. At present, she simply ignored them. She had recently been introduced to the reminiscence therapy group and seemed to be achieving her objective. The idea was not to make her socially competent, but to enable her to maintain some tenuous links with those around her. Joy had no involvement in the group which was usually conducted by a nurse therapist.

● Problem 8. Emily's personal hygiene was quite poor but this was because of her frailness rather than a lack of interest. She needed help to get to the bath and to get in and out of it, but she was still capable of washing herself. She could not wash her own hair, and refused to use a shower device herself. On occasions, because of her urinary incontinence, she needed extra baths. This was an on-going problem and the staff were not concerned so much with an improvement in the situation but more with maintaining her existing level of ability.

Joy had bathed her once and was able to outline Emily's exact ability. This was well documented in the progress notes. Emily had not been verbally aggressive to her during this proce-

dure, but she had been once she had helped her back to her chair in the ward.

● Problem 15. This had not always been a problem because at one stage it was well under control. The nursing diagnosis had changed because no real recognisable pattern was apparent as Emily's behaviour began to deteriorate. The team had managed to establish a pattern for her which seemed satisfactory. They anticipated a decrease in Emily's ability to maintain continence but at present there had been little change over the past three months.

● Problem 17. Emily had become progressively more frail due to the aging process and her failure to exercise. The physiotherapy department had helped her initially but she had resisted them strenuously and it had been decided that the nursing staff should provide the care required. She was still reviewed monthly by the physiotherapist and this review date coincided with the problem evaluation date on the care plan. Emily was usually abusive towards the therapist and did not enjoy either ankle manipulation or exercise.

Joy and her teacher agreed that this was quite a fair representation of Emily's present situation, though there was an apparent emphasis placed upon the biological aspects of her presentation. Joy felt that the one continuous element in the whole case was not on the care plan despite the fact that it had been evident throughout the whole of the hospitalisation period. This was Emily's verbal, and sometimes physical, aggression. At one stage problem 6 on the care plan was isolated as 'becomes agitated on being approached', but this had apparently been resolved by the staff introducing themselves each time they came into contact with her. The progress notes stated that the problem had been overcome and the objectives of less agitation achieved. The teacher asked Joy if she had investigated this area with the other staff; Joy had done so and together they evaluated the data on the existing maladaptive behaviour.

● Emily seemed to be verbally aggressive towards people with whom she was unfamiliar.
● After a short while she would cease this

behaviour and become calm and approachable.

- Her eyesight was failing and she had great difficulty recognising signs and posters around the ward area.
- She was not abusive towards the regular staff members.
- She became more relaxed if she was allowed to vent her feelings without the interruption of the staff concerned.
- She sometimes became abusive towards other patients but this was becoming less of a problem as she rarely had any contact with them.
- She was usually abusive towards medical and paramedical staff with whom she had intermittent contact.
- Although the regular staff said that they did not adopt any special approach towards her, Joy noticed that they often spoke very quietly to her and usually said who they were.

The teacher asked Joy if she felt that a pattern had developed. Joy felt that Emily was unable to recognise new people in their professional capacity and saw them as a threat to her. Because they did not know her, or at least not very well, they tended to be a little abrupt or brusque with her and this only exacerbated the problem. Emily's abusive behaviour was her way of protecting herself from her lack of orientation and feelings of insecurity.

Next, the teacher asked Joy how this difficulty could be overcome so that both Emily and the staff involved did not fall into the same trap once again. Joy decided that an appropriate inclusion on the care plan was the answer.

Comments

Here is an example of a supervising teacher using a ward teaching programme to create a greater understanding of the learner's practical environment. One of the great problems of the nurse education system is the gap that exists between what is taught in the academic situation, and what is practised in the clinical one. Any opportunity to bridge this gap should be used. Where possible, the supervising teacher and the student's primary nurse should work

together on such programmes so that each develops a greater understanding of the other's work practice.

Joy concluded that Emily's unsatisfied need was security, and that this was due to a lack of orientation. It manifested itself by her becoming abusive and violent when approached by those who used an unfamiliar form of address or who were nervous and reticent in her company. Joy converted this into a nursing diagnosis. She then considered the objective of her care.

In the long term it would be impossible actually to improve on Emily's orientation pattern as it was obvious that her sensory/perceptual abilities were slowly deteriorating. The short-term objective would have to reflect the most that the staff would ever be able to expect of her. In everyone's interests it was necessary to achieve the objective as soon as possible and to maintain that level of behaviour. Emily had to feel safe in the company of those people who cared for her and who would ultimately be responsible for helping her to live the remainder of her life with a degree of dignity and enjoyment. Joy constructed the objective accordingly. Finally, she considered the nursing intervention that would bring about this objective. She felt that the clues to its nature lay in the information she had already collected from the staff themselves, from her observations of Emily and from the progress notes. She outlined her proposals to the teacher who agreed with her. Next, they consulted Staff Nurse Keen who considered the situation carefully and agreed that Joy's work should be included on the care plan. This was carried out at the ward handover when Joy was allowed to express her ideas and the need for change in the company of the other team members and the ward sister (Fig. 12.2).

CARE EFFECTS

Over the next few days, Joy's involvement with Emily was as full as it could be. She adopted the approach strategies she had outlined on the care plan and the problem did not occur again. However, when the review date came, the team decided that the problem should remain on the

Patient Care Plan

Patient name: ..Emily .Graham......   Clinical area: Pinewoods.............

Date	Nursing diagnosis	Patient/nursing objectives	Review date
13/2/91	③ Does not socialise with other patients - sits quietly on her own.	③ To make same input into the reminiscence therapy group from her own memories.	27/2/91
13/2/91	⑧ Cannot bath herself.	⑧ To take a bath every other day.	14/3/91
13/2/91	⑮ Has irregular urinary incontinence pattern.	⑮ Remain continent - check pattern.	14/3/91
13/2/91	⑰ Needs support when walking.	⑰ Does not fall when walking.	14/3/91

Fig. 12.1A   Emily Graham's care plan.

Primary nurse: *Staff Nurse Keen* .... Sheet number: *12* ....

Nursing interventions	Evaluations	Date	Nurse's initials
(3) a) Ensure she attends group each day. b) Sit with the same people. c) Do not lead her but encourage her to make one contribution per session. d) Congratulate her if she talks about herself.			
(8) a) Give support as necessary. b) Encourage her to wash when in bath. c) Wash her hair X2 weekly.			
(5) a) Check each hour. b) Ask her if she needs the toilet every 2/24. c) Refer her to ward signpost for toilet. d) Assist her to the toilet at 0730/1100/1530 and 2100 hrs. e) Update urine chart if there is any change in her usual pattern.			
(7) a) Keep walking frame within reach next to her chair. b) Encourage her to walk around the room. c) Do not let her walk unaided. d) Provide passive physiotherapy to ankles once each 2 hours.			

Fig. 12.1B   Emily Graham's care plan (cont'd).

| 27/2/91 | ⑱ Becomes verbally aggressive when approached in abrupt fashion by 'unfamiliar' people who do not identify themselves. | ⑱ To remain calm when approached. | 19/3/91 |

Fig. 12.2A Emily Graham's care plan inclusion.

⑱
a) Do not approach abruptly.
b) Speak in a relatively soft tone of voice.
c) Introduce yourself.
d) Explain your reason for talking to her.
e) If she becomes abusive do not interrupt.
f) Once she has calmed down, try again
g) Do not react to her abusive behaviour.

Fig. 12.2B Emily Graham's care plan inclusion (cont'd).

care plan for the use of future staff, even though it appeared to have resolved itself through the use of effective intervention.

One month later, Joy had the opportunity to evaluate her care more accurately. A new group of junior learners joined the ward and one was attached to her team. She was given Emily as one of her assigned patients and she followed the required approaches of the care plan perfectly.

Emily's only response was to seem a little puzzled at first but there was no repeat of her abusive behaviour. Other paramedical and medical staff were also made aware of this information and they too followed the guidelines with virtually the same response.

Emily died three months later after a steady and progressive deterioration of her condition. The final evaluation of her care, as given by the nursing staff, revealed that the approaches adopted by Joy during her experience on the ward had enabled the nurses to care for her without any serious breakdowns in the patient–nurse relationship. Even during the final stages of her life, when she was totally incapable of orienting herself and had become confused and bewildered by her environment, she remained calm and relaxed in the company of her nursing team.

Before Joy left the ward she carried out a retrospective nursing audit on her work. She felt that she had been instrumental in bringing about a much needed improvement in Emily's care by her isolation of this fundamental problem and outlined it as one of her most important experiences on the ward.

FINAL COMMENTS

Very often, a nursing diagnosis is concerned with inadequacies in the existing nursing care. People are often unaware of their effect on others and are unable to explain the responses they elicit. The only way that the situation can be rectified is by careful examination of all the facts that surround the behavioural incident, even though they do not appear at first to be relevant. No attempt should be made to assess the information until it has all been collected. Only then can obviously irrelevant data be discarded, and only

after due consideration has been given to its overall effect. This analysis usually produces a very simple and straightforward answer to the situation, because in many respects the interaction between two people is often in itself quite simple. It is usually a question of selecting the most appropriate stimulus to produce the required response.

With elderly and infirm people, heavily burdened by the effects of organic brain syndromes, it is too much to expect any real upswing in their ability to lead independent lives. The nurse needs to establish objectives which will enable the individual to adapt favourably to his present situation. This usually means that the nurse must also adapt to the patient. Having made the nursing diagnosis and established a realistic objective, this attitude is then reflected in the approaches laid down for the nursing intervention. Very often, when these objectives are written they seem so obvious that the nurse may wonder if they are not too simple. This, however, is probably why they will be successful, because they will enable the patient to live – and eventually die – with dignity and equanimity. In effect, the process becomes an analysis of one individual's innate responses to another individual and the reciprocation of that response. The nursing process is the ideal framework not only for providing effective patient care but also for creating self-awareness in the people who provide it.

SUGGESTED READING

Oliver S, Redfern S J 1991 Interpersonal communication between nurses and elderly patients: refinement of an observational schedule. Journal of Advanced Nursing 16: 30–38

Ward-Griffin C, Bramwell L 1990 The congruence of elderly client and nurse perceptions of the client's self-care agency. Journal of Advanced Nursing 15: 1070–1077

Ward M F 1986 Constance: an elderly lady. In: Learning to care on the psychiatric ward. Hodder and Stoughton, Sevenoaks

SECTION 3
Professional approach

13

The management of the nursing process

INTRODUCTION

The nursing process is more than simply a method of delivering nursing care. In military terms, the process itself represents the front line of an army in battle and, like all front line troops, it needs a massive support group to keep it functioning at its peak. In theatrical terms, the process represents the actors or stage performers, always stealing the limelight but always totally dependent on the hard work of the 'backroom boys'. In short, the nursing process is dependent on the management that goes on behind it: management not only by senior ward staff but also by unit and senior managers. It cannot function without support, guidance and development and the creation of a suitable arena for it. It must be planned and supported by those who intend to use it, those who intend to benefit by it and those who intend to include it in their daily work routine. The hospital is not like a sausage machine. When a patient leaves hospital equipped with new hope, ideas and faith in himself, it will be because the full panoply of nursing management strategies has acted upon the system providing his nursing care, resulting in an efficient and highly skilled approach to individualising his hospitalisation period. It is all very well having a philosophy of nursing, but without the knowledge of how to make it work, it is as useless as a fully equipped ward without nurses to staff it.

This chapter will consider the effect of the management of the nursing process on both the ward staff and on the patient. Good and bad results of effective and ineffective management styles will be considered. The chapter is divided into five sections:

1. The role of the nurse manager in relation to the nursing process.
2. How the manager can be helped by the nursing process.
3. The effects of the manager on the implementation and continued usage of the nursing process.
4. The responsibilities of the senior and trained staff on the ward.
5. The responsibilities of the patient towards the management of his own nursing process.

THE ROLE OF THE NURSE MANAGER

Inherent in the nursing process is a management element which cannot be ignored, i.e. how to present the process in a package which is effective as well as acceptable to patients and staff alike. Ultimately, control and supervision of this component is in the hands of those responsible for ensuring nursing standards – the middle or line manager. The style and skill of the manager will determine whether or not the process is successful, and the leadership qualities of the manager will be one of the most important factors in determining the degree of success. No matter how well motivated or keen the senior ward staff are to initiate new ideas and technology on their wards, without the support of their nursing officer their efforts can be only partly successful. If he is half-hearted in his leadership or is disinterested, this will be soul-destroying for his wards. At best, it will be a struggle for them to achieve anything; at worst they may give up the fight. The decrease in morale will be felt by the patients themselves and the standard of their care will deteriorate. Every nurse needs to feel that she has some degree of control over what takes place in the ward, no matter how small that control may be. Without a benevolent and enlightened form of leadership, the fight for control can develop into outright rebellion. This, too, cannot be good for patient care. Without the cooperation of the nursing officers and senior clinical specialists, or even directors of nursing services, the support at grass root level for innovative ideas will flounder and such schemes as the nursing process will become impossible to implement.

In psychiatry, where traditionally there is less formality within the nursing hierarchy, this may present less of a problem than in some other, more structured disciplines within the nursing profession (Scott 1982). The communication channels both upwards and downwards are far more accessible to all grades of staff and, consequently, there tends to be a greater degree of equality and autonomy. This allows the manager to gain more insight into the functional needs of his staff and he is more in touch with their methodology and practical involvements. The psychiatric discipline lends itself to active participation by the nursing officer in the nursing techniques and strategies adopted by his staff. Thus the stage is set for him, where good industrial relations already exist, to exert his influence in the introduction of the nursing process, and his knowledge and enthusiasm can add a keenness and excitement to its growth. Let us consider the parts he must play.

LIAISON

The nursing manager must act as a link between his ward staff and their associated disciplines, as well as voluntary organisations and support groups connected with the patients and the clinical areas. It is his job to ensure that resources and facilities are coordinated to provide a potentially dynamic situation for the patient on admission. He must also see that objectives set for the patient are common to all the groups concerned with the patient's eventual recovery. If that cannot be achieved he must at least endeavour to make the objectives complementary. This means he must have clinical involvement and not simply act as an administrator. If he allows himself to become too aloof from the clinical situation, he will be unable to understand the requirements of the nurses and patients and this will be resented.

INNOVATION

The manager's knowledge and understanding of the clinical scene will be influenced by his involvement in it, but he must not become just another 'pair of hands'. He must be seen and recognised as a teacher, without encroaching too much on the domains of the senior ward staff. The only way he can do this is by being one step ahead. He must be creative in his approach and offer new methods of tackling difficult and recurring problems. He must read his subject extensively and be able to apply new concepts to the ward situation. He must be able to advise his nurses on patient allocation, methods of documentation and time structure.

CLINICAL SPECIALISATION

If the nurse manager is to be recognised by his clinical teams as an innovator and developer, he must also show that he himself can do what he advises others to do. It has long been a stumbling block within the nursing profession that when promotion is gained, patient contact is left behind. The advent of the nursing process reverses this procedure, because all activities carried out with patients are considered to be significant, so that none are classed as second-rate or mundane, and the introduction of a specialist into the arena is a necessity. Who is better suited to this role than the nurse manager? Another advantage of this arrangement is that with the manager working alongside his staff, they can see his enthusiasm and support, and feel that he is sharing their experiences with them. This can greatly enhance job satisfaction. The nurse manager may be a senior grade sister or charge nurse who acts either as a clinical specialist or as a coordinator for a group of clinical areas.

INFORMATION SOURCE

Through clinical involvement and liaison with other disciplines, including the education faculty, the nursing manager should develop a body of scientific knowledge which he is in an ideal position to pass on to his staff. If he takes an active role in the meetings of a nursing process advisory group or committee, he has the opportunity of comparing the difficulties and problems experienced by his own teams with those of other clinical areas. By assessing alternative approaches, he should be able to offer his own teams data which enables them to function more effectively and without the associated trauma of the trial-and-error approach to problem solving that they might otherwise have to adopt. If the nurse in the ward knows that her nursing manager is not only able to understand her difficulties but also offer some form of enlightened assistance, her confidence in the management structure will be increased.

TEAM REPRESENTATION

The manager must represent his nursing teams at related meetings and on committees. If, through his involvement, he is aware both of the working situation and the methods adopted by the nurses to deliver their skills, he will give those nursing teams far more credibility. The reason for this is clear. People consider that the representative of a group is exactly that – he exemplifies those he represents. If he is a keen, enthusiastic and involved individual, that is how his group will be thought of. For nursing teams using the nursing process, it is important that they be recognised as scientific and professional, because this will be reflected in the approach used by other professionals in their communications with them. Adequate recognition is a necessary reward for one's efforts.

It will be seen that the functions of the nurse manager in relation to nursing process actions are interrelated with existing managerial activities. However, the nurse manager's more significant role is that of innovator and developer, because these qualities are the essence of the leadership required to manage the implementation and on-going changing pattern of the nursing process and the way it is used and incorporated into other more advanced techniques. It may be more important for the manager to devise new ideas and more effective strategies than to encourage people to work harder. The morale-boosting effect of a professional teacher on those nursing staff who look to him for their lead may thereby be enhanced to produce a more cohesive and coordinated approach towards nursing process activities.

HOW DOES THE PROCESS AID THE MANAGER?

As the manager acts to facilitate the use and efficiency of the nursing process, so, in theory, the process offers him a reward for his efforts. For each individual manager involved in his own particular way there will be different forms of pay-off and reinforcement. These rewards may be the interactions he has with both patients and staff on a personal level; they may be related to the increase in patient and clinical contact that he experiences; or they may centre around his search for an understanding of the basis of nursing activity. However, it is possible to isolate seven areas that might be affected by his participative management of the process.

COMMUNICATIONS LINK

No manager can function without an intimate knowledge of what is happening in his departments. That information is called feed-back and it represents a description of current events vital to his ability to make accurate decisions. Communication in both directions is facilitated by the process, because the nurse must document all changes that take place in the patient's presentation and the type of care and objectives planned by the patient and the team in relation to those changes. The nurse manager has direct access to this documentation and can in a very short time acquaint himself with what is happening, why and for what purpose. In return, he can offer advice, criticism and guidance based on a critical analysis of the situation as a less involved observer, or at least as a non-participant observer. Communication is so important because it passes on knowledge to all concerned and reduces suspicion, thus increasing confidence and a feeling of security.

KNOWLEDGE OF STAFF ACTIONS

It mentioned above, being aware of, or actually participating in, the clinical function of a ward, gives the nurse manager a greater understanding of the complexities of a problem. He is in a better position to analyse situations and make decisions which take into account the various influences at work on those involved. He is also unlikely to ask his staff to carry out actions which are unrealistic or incompatible with their current practice.

KNOWLEDGE OF STAFFING LEVELS

If the nurse manager has the opportunity to compare care plans with the staffing levels that exist in a clinical area, it will give him some idea of each nurse's work load. If one of his managerial responsibilities is ensuring adequate staffing levels in his clinical areas, and he is required to manipulate those staff to get an even balance, any guidance as to staffing needs is of value to him. Morath et al (1990) suggest that being able to identify the different needs of clients might be one way of establishing scheduling and staffing systems.

PLANNING POTENTIAL

In relation to the monitoring of staffing levels, if the manager can correlate the necessary actions and activities of nurses with their effectiveness and adjust the nurse–patient ratios in accordance with his findings, he is in a position to plan new ideas, therapy approaches, etc. He will know whether staffing levels are adequate or whether he needs to seek extra staff from his senior manager. If the latter, he also has the evidence of staff actions at his disposal to present as part of his case. The well-prepared manager who obviously has done his homework has a much greater chance of success than the one who is disorganised in his approach. Because so much information is recorded in documents by the nurse, and a systematic approach is adopted to deliver care, the planning potential offered to the nursing officer is almost limitless (Brooks & Rutter 1990).

BOOSTING MORALE

The nurse manager may influence morale, but if through his involvement in the nursing function he can actually raise morale, the benefits are enormous. Highly motivated staff are far more likely to produce good results and high quality nursing interventions, be prepared to tackle new and difficult problems, and succeed in whatever it is they are involved in. If it is the introduction of the nursing process that has kindled this improved motivation, and the nurse manager has generated enthusiasm and interest as the process progresses, he will find that the number of managerial decisions he has to make in that clinical area will decrease. Disciplinary activity should be practically negligible because nurses are less inclined to be late, get angry or refuse to cooperate if they are interested in what they are doing. Through his involvement in the nursing process, his job as a manager will thus become much easier.

INCREASED STAFF COMMITMENT

This is directly linked to the morale of the nursing staff. If they are involved in their work and feel that they have some degree of responsibility and control over what they are doing, they are more likely to give their best and are less likely to stay away from work for minor ailments. So much time is lost in both industry and the public health sectors because of time off through sickness – and much of that is for single day absence – that any reduction in this is desirable. For the manager, it means that his staffing levels are more likely to be maintained close to the paper quotas, and his planning ability greatly increased.

STAFF EVALUATION

With so much commitment in terms of work hours and personal contact to the clinical set-up, it would be foolish to assume that all staff will respond to the nurse manager in the same way. Individual differences, in ability, potential and attitude, will determine whether or not nurses are prepared readily to adapt to the kind of political environment that the nursing process and the nurse manager create. The manager must know how his staff are functioning and how effective they are in their current roles. He has several different approaches at his disposal. Firstly, staff appraisals can be carried out once a year to establish how an individual staff member is coping with her job. The nursing process allows the manager the opportunity to examine the practical activities of that nurse, and his involvement in the clinical setting gives him insight into how the nurse applies herself to the interactions she designs. Secondly, he can carry out research into nursing functions or construct a nursing audit which will enable him to measure his staff's professional actions (Smith 1989). He must find out how staff function in relation to the process and how effective they are in doing what they say they are going to do. Finally, he can produce criteria sheets which clearly identify areas of action that nurses must follow to comply with the process approach. Obviously, this method must be closely linked to the current documentation in service on his units. He must find a method of monitoring these activities so that he is seen as helping the nurses, not just looking for a method of gaining information about them for disciplinary purposes.

NURSE MANAGER EFFECTIVENESS

As discussed above, the competence of the line manager is one of the principal determining factors in the successful implementation of the nursing process. His role in relation to the success or failure of the process has already been examined, together with some of the ways by which he may benefit from its use. We will now consider how the nurse manager can identify those areas that he can influence and how he might influence them. If staff members are keen and willing, and especially if good lines of communication exist, this task presents little difficulty. This, however, is not always the case. The manager must make himself aware of what is taking place on his wards and he cannot do this from behind a desk or by confining himself to administrative commitments. Total involvement is the most effective solution.

The man whose leadership style is either too

strict or uncompromising or who is unwilling to make decisions because he wants to be liked by everyone is likely to be a bad nurse manager. The process itself, by its very nature, has to adapt to any given situation, and built-in to the system are numerous options for both patient and nurse alike. If the manager is not equally adaptive, then his leadership becomes inappropriate and consequently ineffective. Equally, if he is not prepared to make decisions either about implementation of the process or about on-going difficulties related to it, he will be of no value to those seeking advice and leadership. The nursing process is about people making decisions: it is not possible for it to function on 'ifs and buts'.

It may be difficult for the manager to develop a leadership style within a relatively rigid system such as that of a health service, but certainly it is made much easier for him if he adopts the principles of systematically provided care. By his involvement and professional interest, he can allow others to develop, thus removing some of the pressures inherent in all management – those of responsibility. A good manager therefore allows development and creativity, offers autonomy to juniors, communicates well with those both above and below him, but still retains overall control. The key words here are creativity and control. The two do not always go together. If a manager uses both approaches, he will use the management and clinical tools available to him to best advantage; he will be one step ahead but always prepared to listen to others.

In nursing today, a growing number of people are becoming specialists in very small and limited areas. Such individuals represent an elite in any structure. However, it does not follow that the nurse manager must also adopt the attitude of a specialist. In fact, the nursing process will not allow him to do so. He must, rather, be prepared to take the technology used by the specialists and adapt it for the general use of all his staff in whatever aspect of the psychiatric discipline they are engaged in. To illustrate this idea, four separate areas will be considered:

- nursing professionalism
- nursing research
- nursing and computers
- nursing politics.

NURSING PROFESSIONALISM

Professionalism is the ability to act from a sound basis of knowledge in a systematic and problem-solving fashion. More importantly, most professions work on an independent basis with strict internal control over their own actions and activities. The nurse manager has to collect information from the professional organisations related to medicine and compare their approaches with those, say, of industry. His conclusions should help him to formulate ideas about how best to present nursing to his patients, and he can present himself to his nurses in the same light. He has to determine methods of ensuring his staff achieve professional standards without jeopardising the individuality of the care they provide and, in terms of the nursing process, he must formulate plans for combining new technology with traditional and personal skills. In short, the nurse manager is trying to make nurses more aware of themselves and of the effect they have on their patients, and to give them pride and satisfaction in doing their job well. In this sense, doing the job well is seen as making the patient independent of the nurse, not dependent upon her, and allowing the general public a greater insight into the changing role of the nurse (Pearson 1983).

NURSING RESEARCH

Research is mentioned several times throughout this book, and rightly so, because without proof of actions or justification for action, the nurse remains unprofessional and open to allegations of 'unskilled' or 'haphazard' nursing (Wolgin 1990). The nurse manager, when advocating the use of the process or similar forms of health care delivery, must first consider the research carried out by other nurses and evaluate its implications for his own clinical areas (Fitzpatrick et al 1990). When a new approach is initiated, he must institute his own research using his own staff to validate their own actions, and when his staff have settled down to the new approach, he must carry out continuous investigations to establish whether the system works or needs modification. Being aware of the work of other researchers is the most important factor here, because in this way the nurse manager is bringing scientific knowledge to his unit. The only way this information can be tested is if the nurses adopt the same approach themselves and see what happens. Nursing research cannot simply be discounted because an individual feels a method is wrong, he has got to get out there and prove that it is wrong or, indeed, that it is right. The process, by virtue of its structure, enables the manager to use any number of research approaches because it offers a constant element in a changing situation – something that all researchers require.

Walton (1986) considered the research carried out into the developments of the nursing process and concluded that some research was biased towards the process because it used tools and measures that were based primarily upon the process itself. Managers must ensure that when using the nursing process as a research method, they do not necessarily explore nursing process issues. After all, the nursing process is nursing, therefore it cannot be used to prove the worth of itself. The process should be used to examine factors from a wider clinical context, such as staffing, quality and performance.

NURSING AND COMPUTERS

Most technological advances in the last few years can be attributed to the invention of the microchip, and the technology used by nurses is no exception. The computer uses logical sequences to do several basic functions; this in itself is not outstanding, but the speed of the computer and the quantity of work that it completes makes it very valuable. The nurse manager, like other managers, must use the vast storage and retrieval systems that computers offer (Hargadon 1982) as well as the calculative resources that would otherwise be denied him. As early as 1967, Price looked at ways in which the nurse can use the computer, but where the nursing process is concerned the manager also has a distinctive role to play.

Computer aided care planning (CACP) enables the manager to take an active part in the analysis of care activities, partly because of the way it is produced and partly because of the amount of information that is generated and stored by such systems. The FIP system (1991) described in Chapter 6 contains so many advantages for the care manager that it is difficult to understand why CACP is not used more widely. Consider the features that the nursing process, in conjunction with this modern care planning system, can provide.

- Care plans can be produced as and when they are needed. More significantly, they can be altered and printed very rapidly, thus allowing the manager access to his care teams' work at a moment's notice.
- Reports about patient care can be generated without having to interrupt the clinical staff's activities. The reports can show what changes have been made in a care programme, who made them and for what reason. They can also show the whole care profile of a patient throughout his/her stay in hospital.
- Such work reports can be used to assess the workload of individual nurses or care teams, but the system will also generate information for manpower planning.
- Staffing levels can be calculated from the workload information.
- Evaluations and audits can be carried out from the report writing facilities, which could lead to improved quality of care for the patient.
- Speed, time evaluations and efficiencies can be improved using the data contained within the programme. Managers can look at problems or interventions which regularly appear on care plans and these can be placed in a more accessible library, thus reducing the time it takes to prepare certain care plans.
- Graphs can be generated to show how certain items within the programme are performing.
- Staff development and educational activities can be generated from within the package, in terms of both keyboard skills and the production and analysis of care plans.

The manager can also influence the quality of communication that his care teams have about each other. For example, the FIP system has the facility to make lists of primary nurses and responsible medical staff. These libraries are accessed by the nurses constructing care plans, who thus obtain up-to-date knowledge about the key personnel working within their area. This is often invaluable for new staff members, and particularly for students who may not be able to remember who everyone is without some form of prompt. The manager simply ensures that the libraries are kept active.

The nurse and the manager should be able to use CACP systems for their mutual advantage, as ultimately the patient will be the main beneficiary for the resultant increase in efficiency of the care planning process.

NURSING POLITICS

Nursing is such an intricate and interwoven occupation that a high degree of political involvement is inevitable. Such internal politics are far less marked in psychiatric nursing where hierarchical barriers are less clearly defined (Bellamy 1983) but they do still exist. The use of the process should reduce some of the political agitation by clearly defining roles, but without increasing power differentials, as each nurse is offered some element of control. The process also breaks down some of the professional barriers that exist between the nurse and the psychiatric patient: this will be discussed later in the chapter. Just as important, however, is the presentation of nursing to other disciplines, and here again politics is involved.

It has already been said that most professions have a far greater degree of autonomy and self-determination than is the case in nursing. Many nurses are still finding that other disciplines have more influence over their nursing actions than they do themselves. There should only be one group of people responsible for producing and delivering nursing interventions, and those people are nurses. By implementing the nursing process, the manager can show written evidence of professional actions and judgements of his staff and bring about a greater degree of control for the nurse. Obviously, the interlinking of medical,

nursing and rehabilitative approaches in a treatment programme must be of concern to all those involved, but, just as the doctor makes medical decisions, so the nurse must decide on the complementary nursing care. This is a political as well as a professional argument and cannot be avoided by the manager who believes in nursing progress, individualised care and nursing self-direction.

WARD STAFF MANAGEMENT RESPONSIBILITY

The role of the senior ward staff in the implementation of the process has already been discussed (Chs. 3 and 8). This section further examines their attitude and general approach.

The ward staff management are crucial to the success of the whole system, for without their involvement in new ideas and their willingness to use planned methods of providing patient care, it would be almost impossible for changes to take place. Where a rigid hierarchical system does not exist in a clinical area but where people are aware of their responsibilities and position, a far greater potential for growth exists. Senior staff must be prepared to be wrong from time to time if they are to be respected by their juniors and seniors alike. They must listen to all suggestions and proposals offered by their staff and, if necessary, act upon them, even if they feel that they are not altogether the correct alternatives. Very often, this approach to problem solving gives rise to a credible answer that may otherwise have been stifled had a more traditional approach been adopted. Any period of change involves considerable stress and anxiety for all concerned, but that stress can be reduced if it is shared. Very often, junior, unqualified or learner nurses who are new to a particular clinical scene can see more clearly what is wrong by their lack of involvement in it. If the sister or charge nurse ignores their suggestions because she is too subjectively entangled in the problem, she will cause frustration and resentment in her staff. This may be manifested in their lack of cooperation with her ideas and this will be transmitted to the patient group who will receive a reduced quality of care as a result. It is no longer acceptable to justify a method of care saying that it has always been done this way. Young nurses, in particular today, are far more aware of the failings of their superiors and are in a much better position through their studies to be able to do something about it. The rigid authoritative senior nurse may think that her ward is functioning well, but if she cannot provide objectives for patient care, rationale for nursing action and a systematic approach to delivering care, she will be sorely lacking in her leadership. Her junior staff will have already outlined her failing in their own minds and at the slightest opportunity will attempt to 'do their own thing'. This will create feelings of insecurity and suspicion in the charge nurse or sister who may become yet more rigid and repressive. Open-mindedness is thus the order of the day.

It is not difficult to see why people become set in their ways. A routine offers safety and security and any change may be seen as a threat to this confidence. Psychiatric nurses observe this for themselves when they clumsily attempt to re-socialise institutionalised continuing care patients. However, this situation may be overcome by:

- Communication between senior and junior staff about the changing needs of the staff on the ward in relation to the needs of the patients and the way they are met.
- Consideration of modern methods of dealing with the needs of both staff and patients in a clinical area.

Of course, the senior nurses must be prepared to try out these ideas, not simply talk about them, and, having decided on a course of action, they must then communicate their ideas to senior management to gain their support for proposals. The line manager may be too slow or too immovable to realise new potential or new needs. However, even if support is not forthcoming, or is lukewarm, the charge nurse should at least give the ideas a try (Green 1983). Often, once a new approach has been agreed upon and is seen to be working well, those lingering in the wings will be prepared to join in and help where they can.

Ultimately, the staff owe it to their patients to attempt to do their best for them.

When the nursing process is implemented and in situ and appears to be working well, it is time for the senior staff to consider ways of trimming the system, or improving on efficiency and effectiveness. They must use the system to everyone's advantage. Dick & Foust (1990) outlined a proposal to increase or introduce nursing rounds into a clinical area. The idea is suited to a nursing process format where team nursing is used, because it makes the senior nurse aware of what is going on without formal handovers or reports. It also reduces the amount of time the team spend in conference over the work load because they get advice and the opportunity to discuss the cases with the senior nurse. If more formal handovers are used, then it might be good for the team leaders to hand over their work load to the oncoming shift in the company of the senior nurse, rather than the senior nurse herself passing on second-hand information. In both these approaches, it will be seen that despite the senior nurse handing over responsibility, she still retains overall control. In this way, the senior nurse has more freedom of action. She can decide to act as a resource unit for her staff or become actively involved in some of the more intricate and complex programmes being undertaken by her teams. Her ability to act in a supervisory capacity is greatly increased and she might also act as a back-up system to her junior staff, being available for planning and implementation in their absence.

It is also possible, through this added clinical role, to extend the facilities of the nursing care plan to other disciplines, e.g. occupational therapists, physiotherapists, psychologists, etc., so that they can be discussed in terms of the multi-disciplinary team's overall approach. The nurse on the ward must have total control of the nursing functions on the ward and initiate any and all interventions appropriate to patient care, but she must take into consideration the input from all other support staff. By involving other co-workers in this way, it is probable that there will be an increase in reciprocal communication, and staff will become more aware of what other members of the team are doing. Nurses will develop a greater understanding of the various therapies offered to the patient and will be in a much better position to advise and guide him.

Nurses must remember, however, that often it is just as important to the patient that she provide the incentive for the patient to attend other therapies as provide the actual therapy itself. The senior nurse may decide to function in this way, creating decision-making opportunities for her patients rather than being totally involved and perhaps making these decisions herself on behalf of the patients.

Above all, it is important that whatever type of leadership the senior nurses adopt, they must not allow themselves to become complacent about their perceived success. They should always be seeking ways of improving the system and even if they can find little wrong with it, which is seldom the case, they should question how else they can expand and develop it (Rawlins 1983). Certainly, change for change's sake is pointlessly disruptive, but senior nurses in a clinical area will always be able to identify elements in the system which are not achieving the success they anticipated. It could be that too much time is spent on paper work or in conference; there could be difficulties in allocation; the patient's involvement in his own care may be less than predicted; audits may be few and far between, or flow charts and assessment criteria inadequate. The more efficient the system becomes under the benevolent guidance of its senior nursing staff, the more confident and professional the nursing teams become; and so the more benefit the patients will derive from their period of hospitalisation.

PATIENT RESPONSIBILITY

Throughout this book the role of the patient in relation to his own care planning has been mentioned. It would be foolish to assume that all psychiatric patients are capable of being involved to any great degree and some, of course, will refuse to have anything at all to do with the planning. This should not deter the psychiatric nurse. She must show that she accepts the patient for what he is and does not scorn or judge him in any

way. He must be offered time to get used to this, because in many cases he will never before have been accepted in such a way. He must not be allowed to become a 'passive onlooker in ward affairs' (Pearce 1979), but an active member of the ward group. If the patient feels, through their actions, that the nursing staff are not interested in what is happening to him as a person, he has but one recourse and that is to exaggerate his behavioural presentation. This may eventually gain some response from the nurse but it is more likely to be an adverse one. It must be made quite clear to him from the beginning that he will be expected to make decisions for himself and that the nurses will guide him without advising him. Psychiatric nurses will already be familiar with this simplification of the clinical counselling technique, but it is worth mentioning it here as a reminder that the same principle applies to the application of nursing process commitments. Not only will the patient be expected to make decisions but also to take the responsibility for acting upon them. In this way, he is offered a degree of independence and self-expression that may both help identify areas of need for the nurse to analyse, and provide experience for the patient to learn from. When these two components are combined at later patient–nurse interactions, the result can only be a much greater understanding of the patient's problem by both parties, and a more insightful approach by the nurse in isolating possible interventions that may be of use. The self-confidence and security gained by the patient through making and carrying out his own decisions can only enhance the care offered by the nurse.

Let us consider the points in the nursing process activity where the patient may decide to exercise some element of management responsibility, and see how the nurse might assist him in his efforts.

OBSERVATION

Observation is an activity carried out by the nurse, but if she is to be accurate in her observation she must involve the patient. During the nursing interview she must outline the role she intends to play and how she will expect the patient to offer information that he feels is relevant to his current situation. She must encourage him, through her willingness to accept him for what he is, and without prejudice to her own feelings, to be honest and frank with her. Above all, she must allow him to express his own hopes and fears and not put words into his mouth. She must ask questions which are open-ended and encourage more enquiring interchanges than straightforward questions. The patient may elect to withdraw from the situation or may even react violently to it, but the nurse must not give up her enquiries but keep trying other methods of approach.

It is important that the patient feels that he is accepted and regarded as a person of worth and that the nurse is interested in him and not simply wanting something from him. What information he decides to give will be proportional to the effort made by the nurse. If he decides to 'tell all', as it were, it will be because he trusts the nurse and feels reasonably confident in her company. A nursing interview cannot be carried out in five minutes, but takes time and careful planning if it is to achieve its aim. If the patient feels he can use the situation as a counselling one, then the nurse has achieved far more than pure information gathering, and the initial phase of the process will develop a more insightful basis for assessment. If, as may be the case with the elderly, confused or disorientated patient, very little information is forthcoming, the nurse must construct situations which will allow the patient to express himself in non-verbal ways. The patient will respond to the nurse if he feels safe in her presence, and this applies to the full range of presentations that might be offered: the acutely disturbed individual will communicate freely if a skilful approach is adopted, as will a frightened obsessional woman will if she feels that she is not being judged or criticised. In short, if the patient decides to make use of the facilities offered by the nurse, it is because he feels both that it is safe to do so and that he may gain help by doing so. Thus, the patient may contribute to the management of his own nursing process, by suppressing or not suppressing information relevant to an accurate appraisal of his personal situation.

While the nurse is carrying out the nursing impression, she must inform the patient of what she is doing. He may feel that, because he is in hospital, people are checking up on him and making copious notes about his actions. He may feel that he is being analysed and compared with others. He is right of course, but the nurse must present this fact to him in a sensitive way and help him to understand that he is free to act as he pleases and that he is not being censured for his actions. Once again, if he does not feel safe, he will act accordingly and the nurse's picture of him will be distorted. Above all, the nurse's actions should be obvious and purposeful and she should be able to justify herself in human terms, not just clinical ones. If the patient is to be fully involved in his own care, it is no use presenting him with a completed package of observations/assessments and planned care to which he has made no contribution, as he will feel cut off and manipulated. Certainly, if that programme is implemented, he will feel less committed to it and will, therefore, not offer the kind of highly motivated response to it that he would do if he had taken part in its planning. Success in such a situation will be attributed to the nurse, not the patient.

ASSESSMENT

The only way that the patient can be involved in his own care is if he is included freely by his nurses. If he has to fight for the right to be heard, his hostility will be counterproductive: he may well be ignored by the nursing team and become even more frustrated and resentful. After the information necessary for assessment has been collected, it must be presented to the patient for his own appraisal. It is at this point that the nurse can gain further insight into the patient's perception of himself. If he distorts the truth or avoids making objective statements, it may be that the ability to overcome his ego defence strategies is limited. If he rationalises or denies the existence of certain behaviour patterns, he may be genuinely unaware of his real difficulties and will need a considerable amount of guidance and support if he is to participate fully in the proceedings. The nurse can help him here by taking the assessment step by step, making sure that the patient makes the comparisons and analyses for himself. Obviously, she must make up her own mind about what she feels she can realistically offer him in the way of support but, remembering that it is unwise to offer advice, she must instead help the patient himself to concentrate on areas of importance and distract him from his own 'red herrings'. Getting him to make definite statements about his behaviour and approaches to problem situations is a most important transitional stage for the nurse, because she is helping him to understand where and how he can be offered the guidance he needs.

In the case of patients too disturbed or disorientated to appreciate their own actions, or where memory is impaired so much that patients are incapable of accepting the information as fact, far more subtle approaches must be used. This does not mean that the nurse cannot ask questions about what the patient thinks, because by doing so she may well get answers that enable her to improve care. The secret, here, is to ask questions which can be easily understood and require little communicative skill to answer correctly. Psychiatric nurses must be aware that the longer they spend in their interactions with their patients, the more interesting they become and, consequently, the more the patient enjoys their company. The patient will then be more inclined to link himself to the reality of a situation than to withdraw into a world of his own.

In short, if the patient is to manage the assessment of himself and his own needs, he must be helped by the nurse to do so, and she must offer him both the time and the opportunity to think through his own ideas. In the end, both parties may need to compromise on what they see as the patient's problems, but that in itself is not a bad thing.

PLANNING

The nurse who has involved her patient in the assessment of his own situation must also include him in the planning of his own care. He may need to be informed as to just what can be offered, but he will certainly have an idea of what he would like to achieve.

Patient objectives

Both nurse and patient must examine the patient's potential but it is best if the nurse can allow the patient to set his own performance goals, both short and long-term. In this way, the patient is instigating his own motivational cycle, and his goals are very personal ones. If it is all set before him as a plan devised by someone else, he is working towards someone else's ideal and the plan loses that element of personalisation and hence some of the motivation necessary to accomplish it. Devising the objectives for nursing intervention is thus one of the major areas of the process which requires patients' individual management, hence the term 'patient objectives' used in the care plan. Even if the patient feels he cannot set his objectives easily, he must be guided into making a decision about his own progress. This may involve the nurse providing a set of alternatives, though she should refrain from giving her own opinion about her expectations of him as these may well influence his choice (Richards & Lambert 1987).

Nursing intervention

The nursing intervention is a slightly different case. Selection of the best possible method of helping the patient achieve his desired goals will ultimately rest with the nurse because she is the technical expert. She knows the effect and possible outcomes of the various methods available, and can identify the suitability of each nursing therapy. However, this does not mean that the patient should be excluded from the decision-making process, for exactly the same reasons as have been outlined in the previous sections.

There are several ways in which he can be included here. Firstly, the nurse may again decide to offer a group of alternative approaches. This is all right if there are several different ways of tackling the same problem.

Where the choice is restricted, a second approach may be adopted. This involves the nurse outlining the kind of activities that would help the patient to make progress. The nurse then asks the patient how he feels she might best assist him in these activities, and between them they decide upon the strategy to be adopted by the nurse. In situations where the choice of alternatives is restricted to one only, this may be the only method open to the nurse to enable the patient to make the decision.

Thirdly, the nurse may ask the patient to discuss any alternatives or ideas he may have with other members of the nursing team and then return after a period for 24 hours with his own choice. In this way, her influence over him can be reduced dramatically. Other colleagues, of course, must be made aware of the role they are to play, and ensure that they too do not make decisions or unduly influence the patient's own problem-solving approach.

A fourth method is to provide the patient with written information about certain commonly used approaches previously prepared by the ward team, outlining what the unit has to offer. The patient then chooses the appropriate method from the list, having had to apply the basic principles to his own peculiar circumstances.

Finally, it may be necessary for the nurse to construct the intervention herself because the patient is either totally unwilling, or incapable of doing it. In this situation – not as common in psychiatry as may be imagined by the unskilled nurse or casual observer – the nurse must try to involve the patient as much as is possible. She must talk the whole thing over with him to show why a certain approach is to be used, so that he understands the reason behind her actions. She should then outline exactly what is to happen. She should ensure that at all the stages through the discussion she asks him his opinion about what she is saying so that at heart he may make a decision about some of the finer points in the programme. Other aspects of the intervention selected must also be carefully outlined, i.e. when it is to be offered, how much is to be offered and when it is not going to be offered. The patient may be able to decide for himself how much intervention he feels he can cope with, bearing in mind

that recovery of any description in psychiatry involves a tremendous amount of effort on the patient's part.

IMPLEMENTATION

Once again, the patient's own expectations of his hospitalisation will directly influence his involvement in his own treatment programme and, more importantly, the nursing input. In Chapter 3 it was recommended that whilst carrying out the nursing interview the patient should be given information by the nurse about the current trend in psychiatric nursing. Many people arrive in hospital expecting nurses to carry out all manner of menial tasks for them. Some still envisage the nurse as a kind of handmaiden and feel that their hospitalisation alone will bring about remarkable changes in their health status. They are unaware of the nurse's influence on their progress and become resentful at her small intrusions into their reasons for failure or limited success. They see the doctor as the healing agent and nurses as merely his support. This attitude is more common amongst older patients and it is not difficult to see why. Nurses have always been depicted as carrying out tasks which are unpleasant or person-orientated. Their possession of scientific knowledge is largely unknown to most of the lay public and their teaching role can often only be understood through careful explanation.

If the nurse has carried out this ground work activity successfully, the patient's management of his own interventions will be much easier for him to execute and some degree of continuity can be achieved between the two people involved. If he recognises the nurse as an autonomous component in his treatment programme, then he is more likely to work with her to achieve common goals. Whilst the care may have been planned together, the intervention has to be achieved by the nurse, and one way she can show her professionalism and the significance of her contribution is in the attitude she adopts towards the patient. If she tries to dominate him, he will become resentful and unwilling to participate. If, however, she allows herself to be dominated and manipulated she will be viewed with indifference and lose therapeutic credibility. The middle way of cooperation and mutual respect should be used at all times. How this is achieved will depend entirely on the personalities of the parties involved and the degree of difficulty related to the achievement of patient goals. The nurse must be prepared to listen to what the patient has to say and not simply dismiss his ideas as either excuses or interference. The patient must be helped to understand the nurse's actions and very often it is not enough just to explain them. Even a demonstration may be insufficient to enlighten the patient. The actual experience of involvement is probably the most effective method. Of course, if the nurse considers that the patient is not accepting adequate responsibility during the implementation phase, she must find out why. A modification of expectations may be necessary, and in many respects the patient's involvement, here, is vital.

EVALUATION

In the context of the nursing process, the team evaluation is a continuous element. It cannot be confined to a single activity because in itself the evaluation is merely a method by which further activities can take place. Self-evaluation is an extremely difficult process, even if guidelines are provided. For the patient immersed in his own recovery phase, it can be fraught with hazard. The nurse's major responsibility, here, is to enable the patient to see clearly all the facts concerning his behaviour and help him to compare this with the behaviour they had mutually agreed he should try to achieve. Both parties must make up their own minds and then compare thoughts, the patient always saying his piece first. It is important that the patient gain as much as possible from this assessment of his progress, because if he feels he has done badly or has failed in any way, he may well opt out of the treatment. If the nurse feels that he has underachieved in some way, she must be careful not to transmit her disappointment to him for the same reason. In both these situations, support from the nurse is vital and may involve a considerable amount of hard work, counselling and confidence boosting.

Equally difficult is the situation where the patient has not been very successful but feels that he has. The nurse, recognising his failure, must somehow find a way of demonstrating it to him without causing harm, so that he does not expect to move on to the next short objective encountering an increasing number of difficulties on the way.

The other situation that sometimes occurs is when the patient feels he has done badly but, in fact, he has been successful. There are, of course, several variations on this theme but in all of them it is necessary for the patient and the nurse to find a point of agreement so that progress can take place. The patient's objectives, if they are constructed correctly, should provide a good starting point, but even then ego defence strategies may hide the true facts from the patient. He must make a realistic statement about his response to nursing intervention because it will reflect his own competence and independence. Should he fail to do so, despite the perseverance of the nurse, the possibility of eventual success is limited.

RELATIVES

It will be noticed that the words 'management and involvement' may be used interchangeably in the context of patient activity. Whenever a patient takes responsibility for some action taken either by himself or those acting on his behalf, he is managing the situation. Were he capable of doing so by himself, he would not have come to the attention of the psychiatric nurse, so he will necessarily need varying degrees of assistance to take this management role. This is the nurse's job. If the nurse is unsuccessful in helping him through the decision-making process, then he will not have derived the benefits intended by his hospitalisation. Hospitalisation must provide more than a mere sanctuary: it must create change – change in the patient, change in those with whom he comes into contact, or change in the situation which has created his problem. The patient who cannot manage some change in the areas that have been mentioned has not been effective and, therefore, when confronted with the same set of circumstances, will not have the knowledge or personal skill to deal with them and will revert to the passive patient role once again.

There are, of course, other people who need to be associated with the change – relatives, friends and the voluntary organisations who work in the psychiatric field – and the management of the process should involve them. Once again, the patient plays an important role because he must accept their commitment and significance. A patient's family, especially those with whom he has a close relationship, form part of his daily circle of acquaintances and are, therefore, often well aware of his difficulties. In many situations, they have as many problems as he has but, through some quirk of fate, are more able to disguise them. In family therapy, for instance, it is often noticed that the child reflects the problems of the parents, but only the child is presented for treatment. The involvement of these close relatives is thus of extreme importance in the planning and implementation of appropriate care. Often, they can provide information that would otherwise be denied the nurse, and they are capable of painting a much clearer picture of the patient's background and pre-morbid history. If they can be persuaded to become an active element in the assessment of the situation, they may be helped in their own approaches to his behaviour. If they are included in the process activity from the beginning, the patient's care can be more realistically oriented. Both patient and relatives will have the opportunity to learn different approaches to the problems that have confronted them, though not necessarily in the same way. Also, some of the responsibility for intervention can be taken from the nurse, giving her more time to spend in other areas. Above all, the patient should be able to see that he is regarded with love and is valued by those for whom he cares the most, giving him greater confidence in the home situation. The sharing of a hospitalisation period can be more beneficial than the hospitalisation itself. Conjoint therapy of this nature is suited to the process because in many cases it brings the real problems of the patient to the fore and allows all parties concerned the opportunity to deal with them.

VOLUNTARY ORGANISATIONS

There are a wealth of voluntary organisations set up to provide guidance and support for psychiatric patients. The majority of them function on a self-help basis and because of this are generally organised by people with similar difficulties to those experienced either by the patient or by his relatives. Often, with their specialist interests, they are better equipped than the nurse to deal with the unique needs of the individual, and their active cooperation whilst the patient is in hospital usually means continued support when he is discharged. This continuity between hospital and community helps staff in both areas to create a more realistic intervention programme, and as the care plans follow the patient on discharge to his community, the gap between the two areas becomes narrower. Should the necessity for rehospitalisation occur, as it often does for one reason or another, then the continued participation of the voluntary organisations in the patient's treatment may help to reduce his length of stay. This is because the process of problem identification is much easier to carry out. It may be that, with repeated re-admissions, all the intricate changes in the need pattern can be ironed out so that future hospitalisation becomes unnecessary (Rowel & Terry 1989).

SUMMARY

The management of the nursing process includes all those who may have an involvement in the process, both from a purely administrative point of view and as active participants. It means that those who have problems to solve, carry the process out, but not by solving someone else's problems in doing so. Each individual must concentrate on his own element within the structure and concentrate on his own commitment. If he is successful in this area, then he provides the support for others to achieve their own objectives. Each member of the team must be aware of his own intentions and the importance of his involvement in the treatment. Management begins with the senior nursing managers guiding, supporting and encouraging their staff in the pursuit of an efficient nursing environment. Senior ward staff must decide on the strategies and roles they are to adopt and develop their skills in those areas. The nursing teams must have a clear picture of their own activities, with a definite plan of action for the delivery of the nursing interventions. Finally, the patient must be taught his own role, that of an active participant in his own treatment, with shared control and self-determination. The inclusion of outside participants, both within the hospital and outside it, increase the possibility of success, and they too have their own specific management functions. The words 'management' and 'involvement' are interchangeable within the context of the nursing process, and it is only through this clear-sighted involvement that the changes required to produce patient independence and staff effectiveness can occur.

REFERENCES

Bellamy P C W 1983 The nursing process: A problem of practical theology. Nursing Times 79(6): 35–46

Brooks J, Rutter L 1990 Management – more than a support. Nursing Times 86(5): 64–65

Dick K, Foust J 1990 Clinical nursing rounds: a model for elder care planning at the bedside. Nursing Administration Quarterly 14(2): 10–12

FIP 1991 Newland House, 139 Hagley Road, Birmingham, England

Fitzpatrick J-J, Wykle M-L, Morris D L 1990 Collaboration in care and research. Archives of Psychiatric Nursing 4(1): 39–42

Green B 1983 Primary nursing in psychiatry. Nursing Times 79(3): 24–28

Hargadon J 1982 Computers in management: living with the V D U. Health and Social Services Journal 92: 433–435, 437

Morath J, Fleischman R, Boggs G 1990 A missing consideration: the psychiatric patient classification for scheduling–staffing systems. Perspectives in Psychiatric Care 25(3/4): 40–47

Pearce T O 1979 Communication in the nursing process: a sociological perspective. Nigerian Nurse 10(3): 40–45

Pearson A 1983 What the public thinks. Nursing Times 79(8): 17–18

Price E 1967 Data processing – present and potential. American Journal of Nursing 67(12): 2558–2564

Rawlins T 1983 Do we really need the process? Nursing Times 79(9): 64

Richards D A, Lambert P 1987 The nursing process: the effects on patient satisfaction with nursing care. Journal of Advanced Nursing 12(2): 559–562

Rowel R-H, Terry R T 1989 Establishing interorganisational arrangements between volunteer community based groups. Health Education (Wash.) 20(5): 52–55

Scott D 1982 Limitations of bureaucracy: A conflict of interest. Nursing Mirror 154(1): Educational Forum vii–viii

Smith T-C 1989 A methodology to monitor professional nursing practice. Journal of Nursing Quality Assurance. 3(3): 7–23

Walton I 1986 The nursing process in perspective. Department of Social Policy and Social Work, University of York, York

Wolgin F J 1990 Perspectives on research. Journal of Nursing and Staff Development 6(3): 151–152

SUGGESTED READING

Fow-Unger E, Newell G, Guilault K 1989 Documentation: communicating professionalism. Nurse Management 20(1): 65–70

Liaschenko J 1989 Changing paradigims within psychiatry: implications for nursing research. Archives of Psychiatric Nursing 3(3): 153–158

Milne D, Thurton N 1986 Making the nursing process work in mental health. Senior Nurse 5(5): 33–34

Nisbet R 1988 Conflict and collaboration: a study of voluntary organisations. In: Stockford D (ed) Integrating care systems: practical perspectives. Longman, Harlow, Ch. 3

14

Nurse education and the nursing process

INTRODUCTION

The nursing process has caused a great deal of stress amongst members of the nursing profession, and for a variety of reasons. The saddest of them all is that some are frightened of a method they do not understand and do not have the means at their disposal to find out about it. It is sad because this does not have to be the case. The process is an educationalists' dream in many respects: a definite and systematic approach to examining problems, with clearly labelled areas that can be inspected and expanded in any number of directions. In practice, of course, it cannot be taught in such an introspective way but at least it is a tangible entity offering immense scope to the teacher.

It is necessary for schools and colleges of nursing to rethink their whole approach to teaching the learner how to nurse; those responsible for continuing education should increase their commitment to teaching the qualified and support staff about the process. Other disciplines also should be made aware of the changes that are taking place through nurses achieving a greater degree of autonomy, and be helped to come to terms with this change in role patterns. Transformations are not brought about by wishful thinking but by hard work, and that is exactly what is required if the traditional approaches in psychiatry of pseudo-policing and task allocation are to be replaced by patient-oriented problem tackling. Teaching the nursing process will,

209

therefore, be considered from three separate angles:

1. attitudinal change
2. basic psychiatric nurse education
3. continuing nurse education.

ATTITUDINAL CHANGE

What is an attitude? Pasquali et al (1981) described it as being a 'verbal or non-verbal stance that reflects innermost convictions'. Attitudes are feelings or values, either conscious or unconscious, that mirror the individual's beliefs regarding right and wrong and are influenced by culture and life experiences. They determine behaviour and are often at variance to those held by other people in the same situation. Pasquali went on to examine six stages in clarifying attitudes in psychiatric nurses, whilst other workers examined nurses' feelings towards mental illness (Peterson 1988, Stewart et al 1990, Sharpe 1990, Siantz 1990). What these and many other authors are saying is that a nurse's attitude will influence her behaviour towards her patient, her colleagues and work situation, and the method adopted to deliver her interventions. It will also affect her professional ethics, her understanding of her role and her level of commitment. For example, if a nurse is trained in hospital A where electro-convulsive therapy is not widely used and then transfers to hospital B where it is an accepted part of the treatment programme for many patients, she may find herself in conflict with her hospital B colleagues. Her belief may be that electro-convulsive therapy is harmful or should be used only where there is deep emotional disturbance. Her new colleagues tell her that it is good for all manner of psychotic behaviour and argue that it always brings about desired change. No matter what evidence they present to her, if her beliefs are strong enough they will not alter, and in fact they may become even more deep-seated.

This is a classic example of a clash of attitudes. On the one hand a nurse has a belief about the use of a type of treatment which is at variance with the belief of another set of nurses who hold the opposite viewpoint. Both are influenced by their education, their professional experience and work situation, and yet they are looking at the same treatment in the same clinical setting. The new nurse in hospital B has several options open to her: she changes her attitude, does not change her attitude and carries on in her hospital despite her views, or leaves altogether. The second of these is the most hazardous alternative because the quality of the care she provides in relation to the treatment is bound to suffer because she does not believe in what she is doing.

Let us consider another example. A nurse who has been exposed only to medical, task-orientated approaches to nursing care joins a unit which uses exclusively nursing process techniques. Is she likely to get enthusiastic, become involved and thoroughly enjoy her work? Unless she is offered some form of re-education, she will more than likely become confused, insecure and hostile towards her job and, in particular, the nursing process. What could happen to her in this unit? She may leave, she may pretend to use the process but never actually become involved, she may find herself being criticised and harassed by her colleagues who may ostracise her eventually. The reason she will find change difficult is because of her attitude and the attitude clash she experiences with her new nursing colleagues. Too much effort has gone into forming her attitude for it to be swept aside simply by changing hospitals. Her attitude is an integral part of her, what she believes in and the way she behaves. Some of the factors which may have a bearing on the strength of her feelings are:

● How long ago she trained as a nurse. The more distant her training is, the more deep-rooted are her ideas about her work.
● Her age. We become more resistant to change the older we get.
● The way in which she was trained. She will always see her training as the right way of doing things because it offers her a tremendous amount of security.
● Her experiences of new techniques. If she has none, how can we expect instant change?

- Whether she has received any continuing education to keep her up-to-date with the changing face of psychiatric nursing or whether she still identifies herself with a 'doing' rather than a facilitating profession.
- Whether she fits in with the team. If she sees herself as an outsider, she will behave as one. This means contradicting the team's views to establish her own autonomy.
- Whether she is confident in her own abilities or lacks self-confidence.
- Her intelligence.
- Her basic personality.

The list is as endless as the influences in her life. The point is that people's attitudes will have a controlling effect on their behaviour even if they are unaware of it, because so much has gone into producing them in the first place. If a nurse were asked to help a person commit suicide, it is unlikely that she would say to herself, 'OK, let's do this well'. If a devout Roman Catholic nurse were asked to care for a girl who had just received a voluntary termination of pregnancy, she would inevitably find it difficult to come to terms with the situation. Similarly, if a young married nurse were asked to deliver care to a man who had admitted to having had sexual intercourse with his own children whilst he was drunk, but was now clinically depressed, her attitude towards him as a person may strongly hinder her ability to help him recover. There is no simple way to enable the nurse to overcome the difficulty she experiences, if, indeed, she recognises the difficulty in the first place. However, just as the quality, approach and commitment of the nurse may be the cause of an attitude clash with her patients, so too the way she plans, delivers and evaluates her care may result in an attitude clash with her colleagues. It becomes, if you like, a question of the traditional approach versus the nursing process approach, or task analysis versus patient orientation. In the mind of the individual practitioner, it may simply be perceived as 'This is the way I have always done it in the past and I don't see why I should change now'.

So, before any formal education takes place,

the nurse must be exposed to situations and events, materials and resources which either force her to re-examine her skills in the light of new ideas, or change her attitude about the way she approaches her work. The situations concerned will be attitudinal influencing factors. They re-create a scene rather than destroy it, and give the nurse the confidence in herself necessary to make changes. Without these situations any amount of remedial education will falter; with them growth will be initiated within the profession. They influence not only the qualified nurse but also the unqualified support and paramedical teams, nurse managers and learners; and their continual usage helps perpetuate a gradual and far smoother acceptance of new ideas. As this chapter is essentially about the nurse educationalists, it is important that we examine those attitudinal influencing factors which can either be initiated from the training departments or in which a major contributing element is education-based. A selection of such factors are discussed below, but it must be borne in mind that each plays its part in specific circumstances and it may be inappropriate to use them in other situations. It should also be remembered that these are areas where the educationalist has a very important role to play. Some nurse managers may feel they can organise themselves without the help of the educational staff. This is folly. The nurse teacher is in the unique position of being able to perceive the difficulties of nursing from both sides. Having been practitioners, they are aware of the practical problems facing hard-worked ward-based nurses, and yet they also have the advantage of being able to assess new ideas and technology to which they have greater access. Trying out new techniques in the relative 'safety' of the nursing college enables them to offer alternatives to the practising staff without the patient coming to any psychological harm. In the following situations it is, therefore, vital for the free flow of information to include the teacher and to gain their advice on educational programmes and curricula which will eventually have an effect on the standard of practice within the clinical area. The situations are discussed under four main headings:

1. Documentary elements
2. Participatory elements
3. Committee elements
4. Innovative elements.

DOCUMENTARY ELEMENTS

Assessment forms

At various stages during the development of new techniques, it becomes necessary to revise the existing assessment forms held by the wards. These should be re-designed so that they follow the nursing process formula; offering nurses the chance to assess patients in a systematic fashion will begin the long re-educational programme without actually changing the pattern of events in the clinical areas.

Procedure charts

Most hospitals have standard procedures for carrying out clinical activities. These should be rewritten in such a way as to show a more patient-oriented approach to delivering the necessary care.

Explanatory information

One of the great problems with changing procedures is that people are unaware of what is expected of them. By producing on-going information which can be distributed to the wards regarding elements of the nursing process, a gradual enlightenment should take place before the actual change occurs. The notes can be developed in a logical sequence to coincide with events taking place throughout the hospital, and can be personalised by outlining practical applications on the specific types of wards to which they are circulated.

Placement based learning menus for students

As part of the basic educational programme for learners, all clinical areas used for student placement should have a learning menu outlining what the students could achieve whilst they are allocated to these areas. These menus should correspond to the nursing process formula, directly influencing both those being taught and those charged with the responsibility of teaching them.

Observational criteria sheets

Each ward should produce its own criteria sheets for observation. These criteria sheets should be constructed to include all elements of the bio-psychosocial approach, thus giving a clear understanding of the individual patient in his total environment. Although the basic approach to observation remains constant in nearly all psychiatric situations, different clinical areas may develop facilities and resources which can enlarge upon the accepted practice of gauging appearance, behaviour and communication (ABC of observation).

PARTICIPATORY ELEMENTS

Joint resource centres

Providing information about the nursing process and its related topics can be centralised or situated on each of the basic units within the hospital. The resource centre may include written texts, books, leaflets and handouts as well as cassette recordings, video tapes and example care programmes. This type of resource centre should always be available to the nurse but it takes a considerable amount of time to develop. Ideally, its content should reflect the identified needs and problems of the people who are going to use it so that is grows in value as the nurses expand their knowledge.

Hospital conferences/seminars

Over recent years it has become the fashion to hold conferences in hospitals and invite 'outsiders' to participate in them. This is quite a costly affair. If the hospital holds regular internal conferences, open to all who wish to attend, and includes input from all levels of management and education as well as from the clinical areas, it can contribute greatly in helping the individual understand his own role in the scheme of events. The educational element here is of great importance because the teacher should be able to pass on information from other hospitals and regions relevant to her own work, thus enabling examinations and comparisons to take place.

Joint education/service projects

This does not mean either clinical teaching or formal continuing education but, rather, educational faculty members working in the clinical area to evaluate new ideas and techniques alongside the practical nurse. They may both learn from each other. Faculty practice may also be part of the student supervisory process, or linked to trained staff preceptor support and mentorship.

Ward meetings

It is vital that education representatives attend ward or unit meetings to gain first-hand information about clinical difficulties and offer advice and assistance where possible. This may well be followed by a joint project as has already been described.

Unit advisory groups

Unit advisory groups, acting for groups of wards and having representatives of both service and educational personnel, can consider the problems faced by the unit as a whole and offer advice and assistance where necessary. They should also have at their disposal information about resources and teaching aids which can be utilised for the benefit of the clinical staff. They do not have to meet as a formal committee but may choose to do so. Their main function is to be available to the practitioner to help solve procedural difficulties.

COMMITTEE ELEMENTS

Many of these committees are inter-linked and the reader should bear in mind that it is not suggested that all the approaches outlined here should be adopted. The object of the exercise is to produce the right political climate in which to develop the nursing process, not convince the nurse that everyone has become involved in committees.

Consultative committee

This is similar to the unit advisory group, but it has a specific responsibility to the nursing process and its development throughout the hospital and meets at regular intervals. It, too, should have representatives at all unit levels, who ideally have a working knowledge of the process. The unit must be informed as to who their representative is and should contact him about implementation difficulties. He can then either deal with the problem from his understanding of the particular local situation or refer it to the committee for formal discussion. There should always be an educational representative on this committee who can pass on new knowledge and ideas to its members as well as use information gained for modifying educational curricula.

Documentation review team

As most hospitals devise documentation for the nursing process themselves, this documentation may have to be monitored as to its suitability and effectiveness.

Ethical committee

As the nursing process involves the nurse in producing written evidence of her care with patients, it may be necessary to examine the documentation for possible areas of controversy. Many medical members of staff feel that the nursing process is designed to give nurses power over elements of care for which they have no training. It is important that this is not reflected in either the care plan statements or the progress notes.

Nursing process review and advisory team

This is primarily set up to examine all literature and information about the process as it comes on to the market. All relevant details are then passed on to the appropriate authority.

Liaison committee

The idea of educational and service personnel meeting at regular intervals to discuss common problems is widespread, and not confined to the nursing process. Such meetings are an ideal arena for sharing information and they often produce results that would be difficult to achieve in any other setting.

Assessors' meetings

Under the system of nurse education currently adopted in the United Kingdom, each nurse must successfully undertake periods of continuous assessment. The people responsible for this assessment are usually the nurses supervising the students. During their meetings, they should discuss areas which relate to nursing process approaches, and they should ensure that the criteria sheets used to grade the learner are constructed using process formulae. The logic, here, is simple in that if the learner is trained to think systematically for examination purposes she will have greater experience of the technique in her everyday nursing activities. For the trained staff, the criteria sheets act as a reminder of the approach that the education departments consider the best method for delivering health care. These documents also reflect the current thinking in psychiatric nurse education for both Project 2000 students and those completing the older 1982 RMN syllabus.

Manpower planning teams

The concept of manpower planning is associated more with large management structures than one single hospital or, indeed, a unit of wards within that hospital. However, it is possible, when using the nursing process, to gain a clearer picture of the manning levels required to successfully staff psychiatric wards, and the team doing this could monitor the activities of unit staff and advise senior management of the action necessary to maintain effective use of nursing resources.

Procedure committee

The procedure documents have already been mentioned but, of course, it requires a multidisciplinary group to construct, monitor and modify them. The influence of the educational staff, here, largely centres around incorporating the ideals of the syllabus into the procedural practice, and again it should reflect the nursing process approach.

Nursing audit committee

In the United States the nursing audit is an accepted fact of professional life. Even in the United Kingdom it is growing in popularity as nurses become more aware of the resultant beneficial effect on their patients. From a legal standpoint, it is vital that nurses document correctly and that they carry out those actions they identify as being necessary. Failure to do so may well be regarded in a court of law as malpractice, and, as judges place so much importance on the written documents of nurses, an internal hospital policy of controlling the nurses' documentation would be useful. For the nurse educator, as part of this team, this provides an opportunity to gauge where problems exist and create remedial educational programmes to correct them (Smith 1989).

INNOVATIVE ELEMENTS
Research group

The need for research was never more urgent for nurses than it is today. It would be dangerous to experiment with new ideas and new technology without researching into their effect on both the nurses and their patients. Lauri (1982) stated that nursing research should try to identify particular areas of nursing practice especially within the framework of the nursing process; and a research group could easily outline a programme to examine these areas within its own hospital. Such research might produce work guidance for both clinical and educational personnel. Of course, a local research group must have access to a wider range of information, so liaison between local groups at either a regional or a local level must be part of its function.

Fact finding group

This is basically the same as the research group except that this group's main function is to gather information from other areas of industry and public sector groups, and experiment with ideas and philosophies not commonly found within the Health Service. This may be seen as one of the separate functions of a researcher, although in many respects it could be used as a stimulant or precipitant to further research within nursing. The nursing process has already been incorporated into other forms of health care that have their roots in industry rather than nursing, whilst the audit itself is derived from the financial world.

Library interest group

It is perhaps a little unfair to expect library staff, in nursing or medical libraries, to sift through the welter of annually published professional journals and extract relevant topics for consumption by nurses. However, if asked, they may well search for titles related to individual topics, but they are only able to do this in the journals that they stock. It is useful for nurses to have access to computer search facilities which will identify relevant articles from a broad spectrum of professional national/international journals. Modern technology has also produced compact disc (CD) search systems. Libraries receive quarterly updated CDs containing data about articles etc in hundreds of different cross-referenced categories. Such systems are invaluable to nurses trying to keep abreast of developments, not just within the nursing process but in all aspects of nurse-related care activities.

Pilot schemes

If a nurse has a new idea or wishes to try out a particular approach, it is absolutely vital that she uses a limited pilot scheme to help her evaluate its effects. Pilot schemes are one way of keeping keen and interested nursing personnel motivated in their work. Nurse teachers get the chance to work alongside these nurse innovators and can learn a great deal from their personal experience. Most hospitals who implement the process, use the pilot scheme on one or two wards to examine its effectiveness and to try out different methods of documentation and administration. These lessons can be passed on to the remainder of the hospital staff so that a smoother transition towards implementing the process throughout the hospital is achieved.

University liaison group

This function can be carried out by a single person. The ideal candidate is a nurse with university experience, and as this is often the nurse teacher, who better is suited to the task? The basic aim of the liaison is to establish in what way the university can help both researchers and practising nurses alike. It may involve the use of vast library resources not normally available to hospital staff, or simple guidance on the best method of tackling a difficult problem. Links between the two establishments are vital to their common growth and progression.

Faculty practice

If education staff are to have any credibility within nursing, it is advisable for them to have some clinical commitments. A small case load of patients, regular shift work on particular wards or even, where possible, a ward that is run by the educational faculty, are three different ways that this can be achieved. If nurses are to believe what nurse teachers tell them, the teachers must be able to demonstrate that their techniques actually work. Simply 'doing as I say' will have less effect than 'doing as I do'. In psychiatry, this type of involvement is often difficult to arrange because of the kind of patients that the nurse has to work with, but such activities as holding insight-directed groups or acting as a team teacher in a primary nursing set-up could be suitable ways of achieving this important role.

BASIC PSYCHIATRIC NURSE EDUCATION

A health care system is only as good as the educational process which produces its nurse. If that educational process is haphazard or fails to reflect the changes taking place in other areas, then the resultant nursing care provided by the learners will be equally ineffective or second-rate. Three significant influences have re-shaped the whole pattern of psychiatric nursing in the United Kingdom.

1.   The holistic approach to nursing: the recognition that the patient is more than a set of symptoms, i.e. he is an individual, responding to his condition in his own unique biopsychosocial way.
2.   Professionalism: the realisation that nurses are no longer just a back-up service for their medical counterparts, but an autonomous body with its own separate and very important role to play.
3.   The nursing process: the introduction of a method of delivering holistic nursing in a planned and systematic fashion incorporating the professional aspect of the practising nurse.

It follows, therefore, that the method used to teach nurses their basic skills must be as well planned and as scientific as the principles it hopes to impart. As a nursing process embodies the principles of holistic nursing and professionalism, it follows that it should be used as the method of teaching and not as the subject taught. Nurse teachers must structure their curriculum so that it follows the same formula as the process, and all the information presented throughout the learners' course must be developed along logical interlinked pathways (Hollingworth 1986). Learners must be able to identify the reasons for giving care as well as acquiring technical skills for delivering it, and they must then be able to evaluate whether or not they have been effective and have enough alternatives at their disposal to modify their approach accordingly. The educational wheel that this creates is outlined in Figure 14.1.

As in all nursing courses, there are two basic

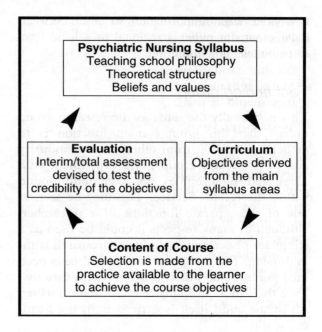

Fig. 14.1   Education wheel.

elements involved in the teaching of psychiatric nurses:

1.   the theoretical context taught in the classroom
2.   the practical supervision of the student in the clinical area.

The two must be realistically linked so that the student can see their interdependence: the faculty must plan the course accordingly.

THEORETICAL CONTEXT

For students in the UK trained prior to Project 2000 developments, the linking of theory to practice was very much the responsibility of tutorial staff. Pre-Project 2000 nurses have access to other staff members such as clinical supervisors, preceptors and mentors to help with this difficult activity. The presentation of the details within the curriculum will ultimately depend on the individual teacher but certain areas must be included in the programme. For instance:

● Basic knowledge of human behaviour both as normal and abnormal responses within a person's environment.

- Observational skills.
- Personal effectiveness and social skills.
- Technical data about treatments, drugs, the law and standard nursing/medical practice.
- Methods of nursing care and the way in which they should be used.

As stated previously, the curriculum must be planned: the subject matter must be mapped out so that not only does the learner know what to expect, but the teacher also knows where his work links in with that of his colleagues. It has been stated that the process should be used as the method of teaching, but during the initial stages of the course the actual skills involved in applying the process should be taught, and in such a way as to make the learner feel involved in the learning process. Individual colleges of nursing will decide whether the information is taught in introductory units, common foundation programmes or in mental health branch programmes of Project 2000. It is important that the right attitudes to delivering nursing care are introduced and strengthened before exposure to traditional medical approaches have made the teacher's job more difficult. Assuming that an integrated teaching programme has been produced with the total involvement of those faculty members responsible for its presentation, we will now consider some of the methods that can be employed to teach the five basic elements of the nursing process: observation, assessment, planning, implementation and evaluation.

OBSERVATIONAL SKILLS

One of the primary functions of the nurse is to make accurate and perceptive observations and then record them in such a way as to be of use to the other members of the ward staff. The nurse needs to gain information of both an overt and a covert nature.

Methodology

Descriptive techniques

Detailed impressions of other members of the student group can be written down, then impres-

sions compared to see the differences that occur. The individual described can tell the group what she considers to be important in her impression of herself, and in this way some priorities for observation can be formulated. It should also help to show nurses that what they consider to be important about other people may sometimes be of little consequence to the individual concerned.

Films/videos/slides

Some form of visual display can be used and learners asked to describe what they see can highlight differences and difficulties. The teacher can also guide the learner in looking for the relevant details and discarding the inconsequential material. Reporting practice here should also begin to strengthen the ability to be precise and concise.

Interactive video

This requires considerable technical support and both computer and video equipment. However, the beauty of this approach is that situations, scenarios and observational vignettes can be replayed and observed according to the individual student's requirements. The interactional nature of the system allows for the student to make decisions concerning the visual images and the computer analyses, and directs the student through an intervention/observational/assessment sequence.

Brainstorming techniques

These can be adapted to the observational process. The members of the group produce a list of everything they saw in a set situation. When the list is complete, they then pick out the elements which are of value and those which are not. This helps to produce observational priorities as well as establishing a group consensus on observations.

Role play

Once again, situations can be enacted for the group to report on. Specific emphasis is placed on the behavioural aspects of the actors. If the participants are briefed well beforehand as to the circumstances leading up to the situation they are enacting, this should also highlight for the observers the difficulties and discrepancies that occur if they do not question people about their behaviour.

Interviewing

Straightforward one-to-one interviews are a good way of practising the skills of eliciting information from people without seeming to interrogate them. The interviews themselves can be videoed and re-run for critical analysis.

Question structuring

Exercises in producing open-ended, non-leading questions for evaluation by other group members will improve skills in both information gathering and the equally important role of counselling and providing psychiatric first aid.

Case study enactment

This is another form of role play except that abnormal behaviour related to specific incidents is introduced into the session.

Experiential techniques

Students are encouraged to explore observational material as it relates to them and to make decisions about what others would say of them if they behaved as they saw others do. In this way, the experiential approach can be used to show that observational material must be verified before it can be regarded as fact.

As the learner progresses through her course, the situations for observation can be made more intricate, and reference to actual situations the learner has been involved in brings an air of realism into the classroom. The various ways that this can be done are discussed later in the chapter. It is important that, as with the technique of brainstorming, no judgements are made about the gathered information until the learner

feels she has enough data to make an overall appraisal of the situation. At that point, the emphasis should switch to the process of assessment.

ASSESSMENT TECHNIQUES

Making a scientific assessment of a patient's situation involves more than simply stating what his problems might be. The nurse must have assessment criteria to work from, and these criteria must be based on knowledge of her own behaviour and the needs of the human being.

Methodology

Producing assessment criteria

Nurses should be asked to produce their own criteria sheets using their knowledge of human needs, activities of daily living, etc. The sheet may be constructed over a period of time and the learner is expected to pick information out of the individual teaching sessions that may relate to assessing the patient. Members of a group can produce either one criteria sheet between them or individual sheets which can be compared and manipulated as necessary.

Assessing their own needs

The next step for the group is to validate their criteria sheets. This is best done by examining their own needs and establishing whether or not the criteria sheets are effective. This has a dual function in that it also makes members of the group think more objectively about their own behaviour. This experiential activity enables the student to personalise the assessment process and makes the decisions arrived at real for each participating member of the group.

Assessing the needs of group members

Applying their criteria sheets to assessing the needs of individual group members may be traumatic for those involved but, once again, it helps the learners to examine themselves more closely.

Once the assessment has been made, the candidates can feed back into the group information related to the effectiveness of their criteria. This may highlight discrepancies which self-analysis had not disclosed.

Assessing the needs of observational subjects

The final test comes when the assessment criteria are applied to data collected from the observational subjects.

PLANNING SKILLS

Methodology

Having collected and analysed data during the observation and assessment stages, the nurse must then learn how to use it. Much time should be spent devising care objectives and relating them to specific nursing functions/procedures and interventions. Obviously the junior learner will have little practical knowledge of these areas, so the sessions should be adjusted accordingly.

Objective criteria

Learners have to find out for themselves the best way to produce objectives that are suitable for individual cases. The guidance offered by the teacher should be in the areas of what constitutes an objective and how to break a long-term objective down into small steps. One of the best methods of achieving this is using a quiz approach. Groups are split into teams; each team is given a set of nursing diagnoses and asked to devise suitable long- and short-term objectives. Points are awarded according to the appropriateness and creativeness of their answers. Time limits are placed on each team and points are lost for failure to beat the clock. This has the added bonus of making the learner work speedily and effectively rather than pondering over every possible alternative. Teachers need to produce some form of 'ready reckoner' for objectives, which shows whether they are suitable or not, so that

the learner can tell at a glance if he has produced an objective or simply an aim.

Mix and match

Nursing interventions are written onto separate pieces of card and the learner is asked to select those that might be useful for dealing with selected conditions and behavioural presentations. This is particularly effective with junior learners, because it also enables them to examine different approaches that might otherwise only become available to them at a later stage in their professional development.

IMPLEMENTATION SKILLS

The classroom is probably the worst place to teach real nursing interventions. Its only saving grace is that it is a 'safe house' for the learner and if she makes mistakes here, at least, she has the chance to rectify them before she enters the real world of the hospital ward.

Methodology

Diagnostic role play

This is role play taken to its logical conclusion. A particular situation is enacted by learners who are called 'participants'. The remainder of the group act as observers. Nursing intervention is offered and when the participants get to a point where they feel they are doing badly or cannot handle the problem, they can stop the action. The participants are then offered advice by the observers and, when the participants feel they have a method of dealing with the difficulty, the action continues. Likewise, the observers can stop the action if they feel that a particular approach is not working. The scenario continues until the problem is dealt with. In this way, nursing intervention is tailored to fit the situation and the experience of working through the problem in a systematic way and eventually gaining an end result should instil enough confidence in the learner to enable her to remain more poised and sure of herself when confronted with patients' problems in a ward.

Video recordings

For those who do not favour experimental learning techniques, there is always the video recorder. Nursing interventions from the clinical area can be shown to groups who critically discuss the implications and effects of what they see.

Case study conference

This is a similar approach to the video presentation except that here the teaching aid is a case study, real or imagined, to illustrate approaches that have been used by other nurses. Once again, the group has to critically discuss what they read.

It may also be helpful to invite primary nurses or mentors from clinical areas to come into the educational department and work for set periods of time on theoretical patient problems similar to those that might occur in their work areas.

EVALUATION SKILLS

The evaluation of one's care can only be done after the care has been offered; in a theoretical situation, the opportunities for evaluation are therefore limited.

Methodology

Evaluation criteria sheets

The learners are asked to compile a list of items that might be used to produce an overall evaluation criteria sheet. These can then be applied to case studies to see if they are acceptable.

Self-analysis techniques

In Chapter 8, self-analysis of nursing care was discussed and the same criteria could be used here for learners involved in role play situations. It is also of value if the learner writes down how she feels about her performance so that this can be discussed in relation to her group's appraisal of her actions.

Total evaluation of nursing process activities

This again can be done by producing either flow charts (Fig. 14.2) or work sheets (Fig. 14.3) which the learner follows through to see how she has done from a systematic point of view.

Each teacher has his or her own particular style of presentation, and the illustrations chosen may not fit in with that style. However, as long as during each of the sessions set aside for skills training, the subject matter dictates the method of teaching, then the learner will benefit from the experience. 'Doing it' is a far more worthwhile experience than 'talking about it'. As the learner becomes more experienced, further variations can be employed to provide her with alternative approaches. Teachers must resist the temptation to put medical diagnoses into little boxes and teach them with the nursing process tagged on at the end for good measure. Sessions devoted to, for example, the aetiology and pathogenesis of 'Hysterical reaction' or 'Schizophrenia' are out of place here because the teacher should instead focus on the behaviour that results from those conditions and plan strategies that might deal with them. The clinical symptoms will be learnt through the teacher's skilful adaptation of observational notes taken by the nurse. These notes are then interpreted to find out why the patient is behaving the way he is. One method of encapsulating every aspect of a condition and its care is the use of the nursing intervention analysis card (Fig. 14.4). These cards are filled in by the learner from case studies or from the information presented by the teacher. They can also be used by the teacher as simple lecture guides. The other important use for these cards is in the clinical area, where they can be used to build up an impression of a particular patient nursed by the learner.

TEACHING AIDS

If the educational department is to provide suitable study facilities for the learner in the area of nursing intervention, certain dual purpose aids must be available. Dual purpose in this instance

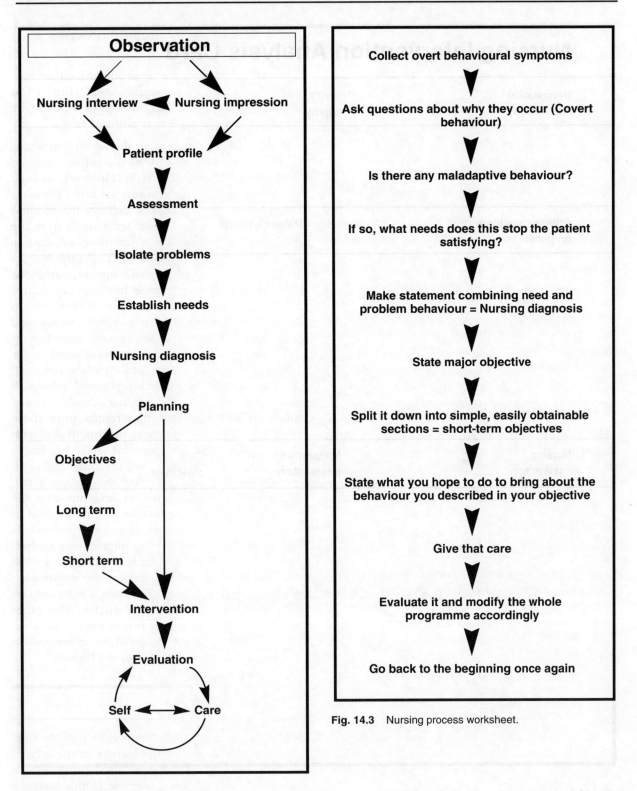

Observation

Nursing interview ← Nursing impression

Patient profile

Assessment

Isolate problems

Establish needs

Nursing diagnosis

Planning

Objectives

Long term

Short term

Intervention

Evaluation

Self ←→ Care

Fig. 14.2   Nursing process flow sheet.

Collect overt behavioural symptoms

Ask questions about why they occur (Covert behaviour)

Is there any maladaptive behaviour?

If so, what needs does this stop the patient satisfying?

Make statement combining need and problem behaviour = Nursing diagnosis

State major objective

Split it down into simple, easily obtainable sections = short-term objectives

State what you hope to do to bring about the behaviour you described in your objective

Give that care

Evaluate it and modify the whole programme accordingly

Go back to the beginning once again

Fig. 14.3   Nursing process worksheet.

Nursing Intervention Analysis Card

Behavioural impression	Patient's strengths	Clinical data

Effects symptoms on patient	Patient's needs	

Nursing intervention	Rationale for intervention	Care objectives

Fig. 14.4 Nursing intervention analysis card.

means that both the faculty and the learner can derive benefit from use of the aids. Obviously, the most useful and basic of these aids is the library. Nursing libraries, where the librarian is constantly researching relevant information and distributes it for the use of the faculty, are an extremely useful asset and provide a valuable source of background material for the learner to incorporate into her own studies. The most up-to-date information, of course, comes from the nursing journals, and inter-loan library facilities should be extended to all the learners so that they can gain access to the large number of reference books published annually. For the teacher, the usual audio-visual materials on the process are essential, but only for the initial learner; all other students should be able to put the principles into practice. For that purpose, the school should set up its own nursing process resources unit.

NURSING PROCESS RESOURCES UNIT

A resource centre should be set up in the school for use by both teachers and faculty staff. It should contain a combination of teaching materials, background information, criteria sheets, work cards, flow charts, etc. Its main function is to have the relevant information and back-up data on any aspect of the nursing process. The following represent some of the contents of a resources unit.

Case studies

These are categorised according to their functional areas. They can be either written or tape recorded. They should provide good background information about the patient and a detailed observation of his behaviour whilst in hospital, especially on admission. They can be written by the faculty or the learners themselves, or can be transcripts of care studies carried out by the learner whilst on ward placement.

Reference data

The photocopying of journal information is illegal so a record must be kept of the relevant articles available. Here, the librarian can be a great help. The articles can be divided into various categories such as:

- assessment methods
- background information
- research
- printed care plans
- standard care plans
- associated topics.

The bibliography must be revised and increased as much as possible if it is to reflect current trends and approaches to the teaching and use of the nursing process.

Documentation

As each hospital will often be using its own adaptation of the basic documentary format, it is essential that the unit carries sufficient stocks to enable learners to familiarise themselves with the documentation.

Care plans

A collection of care plans related to the case studies, completed by either the teachers or the learners, can be used to reinforce the correct way to approach the planning aspect of care. It is always useful to have copies of extremely poor or inadequate care plans for critical appraisal by the learner, though particular care must be taken that these plans are indexed specifically as 'rejects'. Attached to the completed plans could be a summary of the assessment criteria used to produce the plan, the long-term objectives and the rationale behind the care selected.

Video-recorded interviews

Many nurses have great difficulty interviewing patients. The skills of interviewing are complex and related to other aspects of personal interactions, and no two interviews will be the same. However, it is possible to create role-play situations which, when recorded and played to learners, will give some idea of the alternative approaches that are available. Ideally, the recorded interviews should be related to the case studies, so that the learners have some background information about the patient and can understand the rationale for the strategies used. Another useful approach is to show bad interviews as well as good ones, so that the learner can examine what faults are likely to occur and their effects, and discuss ways of avoiding them. Finally, allowing the learners to get involved in interviews, recording them and playing them back, should give learners the opportunity critically to examine their own performances and plan other possibilities for future use. It also allows them to see where their own personal strengths lie so that they can build on them and create their own style of interviewing.

Tape-recorded interviews

These are used in the same way as the video recordings but the learner is, of course, confined to listening to the interview. By doing so, the learner can examine the effects of tonal stimuli and judge whether or how these effects can be used to obtain a better communicative pattern with the patient. Once again, bad interviews should be used as well as good ones, to show how the nurse can be responsible for poor communication by the way she speaks.

Role-play cards

Scenarios of different situations can be written down for role-play activities. Any number of variations can be used so that the learner has the opportunity to experience difficult and unusual as well as commonplace problems.

Peer assessment cards

In any one of the role-play or experiential learning situations that the resource unit produces, the appraisal of a learner's peers may well offer participants new ideas or constructive criticism that can be of benefit at a later stage. It is wrong to assume that the teacher has all the answers; often the group can construct strategies that are far more enlightened or creative. These should

be re-casted for future use. An assessment card can be constructed in such a way as to grade activities in terms of strengths and weaknesses, showing where and why the participant went wrong, and what she can do to rectify her problem, and highlighting areas of success.

As the unit progresses and is gradually enlarged, other useful data and tools can be included. All the information contained within it should be clearly indexed and cross-referenced so that it is easy to use. A record of usage must be kept so that a teacher can see at a glance which exercises or information particular groups have already been exposed to. Case studies should have complete sets of documentation to go with them so that the learner can follow the systematic approach to care from start to finish. For example, a case study of a woman suffering from puerperal psychosis will have the background history and admission notes, observational data initial and on-going plans (and alternatives if necessary to show the diversity of approaches that could be used), medical treatment records and all relevant charts and programmes. If possible, discharge summaries and community psychiatric nurse care plans can also be included to show the natural progression of the care process. Involvement of voluntary organisations and self-help community groups should also be included within the package. In this way, the learner gains a complete picture of a patient's response to her illness and the methods used to teach her how to overcome her difficulties. A method of nurse education that presents psychiatry as fragmented aspects to be tied together, will only perpetuate the traditional method of delivering care, that is care by crisis.

CLINICALLY-BASED TEACHING

Many students of nursing want to get involved with nursing intervention as soon as possible, but this can create problems because all the necessary information required to produce appropriate interventions might not have been obtained. However, no-one would argue that the only place to teach psychiatric nursing is in contact with the patient (Reynolds 1982). The application of skills in a practical setting offers the student the unique opportunity to develop as a nurse in a way that is totally impossible to achieve through purely theoretical systems. More importantly, as Reynolds and Cormack (1982) observed, there is a tendency to teach psychomotor skills in the classroom, but psychiatric nursing is all about interaction and interpersonal skills. These skills can only be acquired through patient contact. It could be argued that the psychomotor aspects of the nurse's role – i.e. the gaining of information, assessing and planning – could be taught in the classroom, whilst the interpersonal skills of nursing intervention and evaluation should be developed in the clinical area. It is important, therefore, that when considering ward-based teaching, the teacher should be prepared to teach within the context of the situation existing at that moment in time, and not relate theory to a contrived and unreal situation.

Very often, the interaction between the teacher and the student in the ward is exactly the same as that which you would expect in the classroom. However, the ward must not be seen as an extension of the classroom but, rather, an area which provides another element in the whole teaching programme. Of course, if the education process is to work, then correct supervision of learners must be available. Students should never carry out nursing actions on their own until they have learnt how to do them properly or are confident enough to be able to ask for help. Even straightforward conversations with patients, group activities and simple counselling sessions should be monitored if any advice, help and guidance is to be offered and learning is to take place. If a nurse is allowed to function independently before she has learnt how to do her job, the chances are she never will learn how to do it. Supervision may be carried out by someone such as an allocated primary nurse, or the team leader in a group of nurses. Senior ward staff should not really be made responsible for the day-to-day supervision of students. The staff nurse grade is the ideal mentor/supervisor, whilst they in turn should be monitored by the senior ward staff.

The teacher's role here is to coordinate these different groups of people to ensure that the student receives the correct amount of supervision, whilst allowing for their personal and professional development.

Below are some ideas that could be used to make clinically applied teaching more interesting, more relevant and more objective. Some of them are already being used extensively; others require time and planning to ensure that they are used ethically, and permission may have to be sought from those involved before implementation takes place.

Patient-centred teaching

Most teachers are aware of the principles of teaching learners the theoretical side of caring for a patient. The next stage is for the student to become involved with the patient's care, his interventions and interpersonal activities. Observations are discussed with the learner so that a clear picture of all the relevant details about both the patient and the learner can emerge – simply going over a patient's signs and symptoms is not patient-centred teaching.

Problem-oriented teaching

As Reynolds and Cormack (1982) pointed out, a problem-oriented approach to psychiatric nurse education is the only way of moulding the educational process to fit the learner's needs. Being in the clinical area with the learner, observing the difficulties she experiences and then helping her to rectify them is the most scientific method of facilitating learning that teachers have at their disposal.

Teaching for change

Students must be trained to identify and report all elements of change in patient behaviour. The student should be taught how to observe change, how to create situations which require change and how to interpret behaviour so that accurate conclusions can be drawn from the change. This education can only be done by supervising situations as they occur and observing the effects of the environment and social patterns at work at that moment in time.

Clinically-based resources

The closer that facilities and resources are to the student, the more chance there is that she will use them. Information that is accessible becomes common knowledge. A resources unit, such as that described earlier in this chapter, might be out of place in a clinical area, but data about social skills, personal effectiveness, and needs theory and its implications may be useful to the student. The teacher must show how the perfected skills of human interactions can be utilised by the nursing process to produce therapeutic and acceptable change.

PLACEMENT INVOLVEMENT

The student involved in psychiatry will, fortunately, be placed in other disciplines during the course of her training, usually during her initial common foundation programme. This has the effect of broadening her interpretation of psychiatric conditions and human behaviour in general. However, the basic principles adhered to in the nursing process apply no matter where she is practising her skills. The teacher must be prepared to follow the student into the various placements and show how interactions that take place there are as valuable as those that occur in the ward. This means that some degree of co-operation must exist between the education faculty and the multi-disciplinary departments. It is vital that the nurse be given the opportunity to examine her role and her approach when she moves from the relatively safe ground of a hospital ward into:

- the community, social services and voluntary organisations
- night duty
- occupational therapy, industrial therapy
- re-settlement services
- child psychiatry, adolescent units
- alcohol, drug dependency units

- mother/baby units
- day centres, mental welfare clinics
- family therapy groups.

It is the teacher's responsibility to supervise the student placements and to show that the basic philosophy of planned and individualised nursing intervention can be successfully delivered irrespective of the professional arena in which it is offered.

The various approaches to clinically-based teaching outlined above will need back-up resources and, in many respects, these are even more important than the supervisory element involved in their application. All of these aids need to be completed, marked or monitored by the learner herself so that they can be used as a written record of events for future discussion or immediate action. They include:

Ward diaries

These are written records of personal events taking place during a learner's placement. They can either be used for consolidation purposes, i.e. on return to the education department they can be discussed in the clinical area with the teacher and supervisory nursing staff; or they can be used to compile role-play situations to discover alternative strategies to those adopted by the learner at the time of writing.

Ward projects/care studies

It must be stressed that these will be a record of the nursing process in operation and represent one patient's involvement with the process. The traditional approach to case studies, which includes medical background, intricate webs of personal data and multi-disciplinary treatment details, are not consistent with the modern concept of a nurse's care study.

Interaction records

Projects related to the relationship between the nurse and a single patient in the clinical area require supervision and patience to prepare. If done correctly, they constitute an invaluable part of the learner's on-going clinical experience.

Assessment booklets

These are written records of the rationale for carrying out nursing interventions which can be examined and analysed after the consequences of the interventions have occurred.

Problem and effect schedules

Once again, these are records of the nursing actions offered by the learner, but here the consequences of those actions are also recorded at a later date. In this way, over a period of time, the learner can get a picture of the effect she has on her patients and, if necessary, seek guidance from both clinical and tutorial staff as to how she might modify it.

Before concluding, it should be said that in addition to receiving adequate supervision from the education faculty, geared towards developing her skills with people, and the appropriate teaching aids, it is vital to the learner that these are followed up by clearly related theoretical information on return to the teaching centre; otherwise a great rift will appear in her overall appreciation of her role. One way of ensuring that this rift does not occur is to have a student consultative group responsible for advising tutorial staff of the changing needs of the learners within the various clinical modules. The information received from this group should not affect the basic curriculum because, if it has been prepared correctly, it will already have an in-built adaptability element. However, the group should increase the communication flow between the learner and the teacher, thus reducing any friction or frustration that may otherwise appear at their professional interface.

CONTINUING NURSE EDUCATION

Nurse education does not stop simply because the nurse has passed her final examinations for registration. It is an on-going process and involves learning about role situations, personal strategies and the right way to get the job done properly. Nurses in the early stages of their staff nurse role need almost as much guidance and supervision as they did as students. This can be provided by other, more qualified, nurses acting in a mentor capacity. However, just what is it that these newly qualified nurses and their mentors need to consider?

Because of the changing pattern of our modern society, the nurse has constantly to be aware of and understand new concepts and their influence on psychiatry and psychiatric patients. If a new or alternative approach to problem tackling presents itself to the nurse, it is her responsibility to find out whether it actually works and, if it does, to adopt it with her patients who expect quality care from her. It is the responsibility of those who teach in continuing education to ensure that a good flow of information about current trends reaches the qualified staff, and in such a way that it can be identified and incorporated into existing nursing patterns without too much upheaval.

At the beginning of this chapter, attitudinal influencing factors were discussed. It was mainly towards the qualified members of the nursing team that these comments were directed, as the more junior trained staff will already have received teaching and information and had the opportunity to practise the process whilst involved in their courses for registration. But what of the qualified sister or charge nurse of 25 years' experience who openly admits that she does not wish to become involved in 'new fangled' ideas? There rests the challenge. If a new idea – in this case the nursing process – has been proven to offer a better standard of care to patients and has both social and professional benefits which make it far more effective than traditional methods, those senior staff should adapt to the new method.

Senior nurses should be offered the process in such a way as not to threaten their position, their pride or their dignity. They must be shown how to use it both effectively and efficiently and, above all, they must be provided with an arena in which to voice their fears without threat of ridicule from their colleagues. And, of course, it is not just the senior trained staff who are the target population for this activity, the nursing aids, care assistants and support staff also need to be given a complete run down on their roles within the system and shown how best to utilise their skills to improve on their performance.

Let us consider some of the methods available to the continuing nurse education team to aid them in this teaching task.

Workshops

These are specifically designed study days which offer both theoretical input and practice/experience facilities. The first participants should be sisters, charge nurses and nursing officers, for ultimately the success of a method of health care delivery will depend on their belief in it. The groups should be small, between 6 and 10 members, allowing for maximum teacher contact. Part of the teaching input should come from senior nurses already using the process so that first-hand knowledge of its practicalities can be examined. The workshop should consist of such items as:

- introduction to individual patient care (IPC)
- the reality of staff/patient allocation
- local documentation usage
- process counselling
- discussions on common problems and methods of overcoming them
- research presentation.

The teacher must provide a variety of aids to the participants so that practical workshop activities can be demonstrated as realistically as possible. Such aids include:

- case studies
- pre-planned care programmes
- allocation sheets
- criteria sheets for assessment
- flow sheets/progress data
- nursing process orientated managerial problems to be worked through in syndicates to a satisfactory conclusion.

Information must be given on the use of the nursing process locally and the participants should be given references to follow up for their own reading after the workshop. Each participant must receive an offer of back-up services to help the implementation procedure.

College/school placement

It is often possible to allow qualified members of staff the opportunity to 'go back to school' by conducting small study blocks for them within the educational department. Groups of 4–6 nurses from the same specialism can be offered time to explore new developments within the curriculum, including use of the nursing process and associated models of nursing, whilst spending some time with the students involved in the same activity (Peplau 1987, de la Cruz 1988, Fruehwirth 1989, Herrick & Goodykoontz 1989). The benefits of such experience are that the nurses not only get the opportunity to use the nursing process as it has evolved within an integrated curriculum, but also to develop ideas and practice within the 'safe' patient-free environment of the educational department.

Inter-hospital exchange

In many parts of the world, the inter-hospital exchange is a popular method of educating trained staff. It involves selected individuals working on an exchange basis with their opposite numbers in hospitals in different parts of the country, so that they can explore alternative methods of tackling similar problems. The period of secondment varies, but several weeks is desirable.

Working lunches

Here, trained staff meet over a buffet lunch to discuss with experienced users of the process, their own difficulties and approaches. This is an ideal and extremely civilised method of maintaining interest and keeping motivation high.

Circulars

Much information is produced both locally and nationally about the nursing process, and this should be collected, correlated and circulated to all the clinical areas. New publications, journal articles and news sheets should be included in the data sheet.

Information centres

A telephone number should be circulated to the wards which puts the enquirer in touch with a link nurse whose sole job is that of coordinating the introduction of the process. This person, usually an experienced sister or charge nurse, should be able either to deal with the query or put the enquirer in touch with someone who can. Nursing process link nurses are also responsible for touring the wards and aiding staff 'on the spot' with the implementation of the process.

Committee liaison

A member of the in-service team must liaise with the various nursing process committees to establish the changing need pattern of the nursing staff. In this way, future workshops, study days and resource facilities can be geared towards solving real problems rather than offering out-of-date information about imagined ones. This is one of the most effective methods of feed-back available to the team.

Ward visiting

The link nurse has a basic responsibility to visit wards for teaching purposes, but the team members should also visit the wards to gain a clear picture of what is required by the nursing staff. As a feed-back method it is invaluable.

Resources unit

In the same way as nurses in training should be offered access to local resource units, so too should the other members of the nursing team. This can be a shared venture with both the library and education faculty providing an input.

Research

The continuing education team should not only conduct their own research, but also encourage sisters, charge nurses, auxiliaries and nursing officers to initiate their own projects. The education department could coordinate the projects, thus ensuring that findings and results are distributed amongst other staff members. The nursing process is an excellent field for research, offering limitless opportunities for the enquiring nurse and nurse educationalists alike.

The continuing or post-basic education team must ensure that they coordinate their education programme and that the participants in their activities receive effective back-up facilities to aid them in their implementation and development of the nursing process. This involves a close liaison with the nurse managers. Many nurses say that they only began to realise what nursing was all about after they became qualified, and, certainly, actually doing the job is the greatest method of education that is available. The continuing education team must make sure that what the nurse learns is the right method and not just the quickest or most cost effective or least time consuming. They must be made aware of the nursing process, its suitability and its effectiveness. Psychiatry needs the process if it is to give patients the opportunity to develop with dignity, and on-going constructive and scientifically oriented education from professionals is the best method of getting the process started.

SUMMARY

This chapter has examined the three areas in which the nurse teacher can play a part in introducing the nursing process to nurse practitioners: the attitudinal influencing area, basic nurse education and continuing education. In all three areas, methods have been outlined which may make the teacher's job more effective. All of them require considerable time and effort in both planning and presentation if they are to succeed, but professional teachers must be prepared to commit themselves to the task if they want to see any change take place within the clinical area. This is the principal point made in this chapter: that teachers should get involved in the process and not just sit on the sidelines and give instructions. Teachers must be seen to be able to practise what they preach, or they will lose their credibility within the profession.

In conclusion, it must be said that it is an extremely imaginative learner nurse who can explore in theory alone alternatives within the scope of the nursing process without ever having used the process in the clinical area. The nursing process is recommended by senior and governing nursing bodies as the most effective method of delivering nursing intervention. It is not just an educational device for students to pass examinations. All clinical areas must adopt the nursing process, and educational staff must encourage their staff to become experts in its usage. Only in this way can the skills of the nurse in psychiatry be enhanced and perpetuated for the benefit of both the patient and the discipline as a whole.

REFERENCES

de la Cruz 1988 In search of psychiatric nursing theory: An application of Oren's self care model's applicability. Canadian Journal of Psychiatric Nursing 29(3): 10–11, 14–16

Fruehwirth S E S 1989 An application of Johnson's Behavioural Model: a case study. Journal of Community Health Nursing 6(2): 61–71

Herrick C A, Goodykoontz L 1989 Neumans system model for nursing practice. Journal of Child and Adolescent Psychiatric and Mental Health Nursing 2(2): 61–67

Hollingworth S 1986 The nursing process: Implications for curriculum planning. Journal of Advanced Nursing 11: 211–216

Lauri S 1982 Development of the nursing process through action research. Journal of Advanced Nursing 7: 301–307

Pasquali E A, Alesi E G, Arnold H M, De Basio N 1981 Mental health nursing. C V Mosby, St Louis

Peplau H E 1987 Interpersonal constructs for nursing practice. Nurse Education Today 7: 201–208

Peterson D 1988 The norms and values held by three groups of nurses concerning psychosocial nursing practice. International Journal of Nursing Studies 25(2): 85–105

Reynolds W 1982 Patient centred teaching: a further role for the psychiatric nurse teacher. Journal of Advanced Nursing 7: 469–475

Reynolds W, Cormack D F S 1982 Clinical teaching: an evaluation of a problem orientated approach to psychiatric nurse education. Journal of Advanced Nursing 7: 231–237

Sharpe T 1990 Unpopular psychiatric patients. Nursing Time 86(8): 65

Siantz M L 1990 Issues facing psychiatric nursing in the 1990s'. Journal of Child and Adolescent Psychiatric Mental Health Nursing 3(2): 65–71

Smith T C 1989 A methodology to monitor professional nursing practice. Journal of Nursing Quality Assurance 3(3): 7–23

Stewart K, Frederick H, Mitchell-Pederson L 1990 Caring for the unwanted patient. Nursing 20(10): 44–48

SUGGESTED READING

Abdullah F 1957 Methods of identifying covert aspects of nursing problems: a key to improved clinical teaching. Nursing Research 6(1): 4–23

Burnard P 1983 Through experience and from experience. Nursing Mirror 156(9): 29–34

Cartwright M 1988 Computers and nursing education in one Australian tertiary institution. Nurse Education Today 8: 23–29

Moss A R 1988 Determinants of patient care: nursing process or nursing attitudes. Journal of Advanced Nursing 13(5): 615–620

Sharpe T 1991 Whose problem? Nursing Times 87(3): 36–38 (Attitudes towards patients with mental health problems)

15

Communication and the nursing process

INTRODUCTION

The nursing process has come to mean different things to different people. For some, it represents the basis of clinical actions; for others, the method of maintaining clinical standards. Teachers use it as a teaching technique, and managers as a method of organising staff and caseloads. Yet others see it as something which, if ignored, will hopefully go away or disappear altogether. This last reaction is not as strange as initially it may seem. The nursing process has a great deal to offer individual nurses, and can transform the settings in which they work and the resources available to them to implement new ideas and technology. However, the nursing process cannot hope to be all things to all people. It does not solve all the problems of the psychiatric nurse, manager or teacher. It cannot offer a solution to staff shortages, lack of finance or social support. Above all, it will never solve the problem of psychiatry itself – yet herein lies a clue as to just what it does have to offer.

The presentation of psychiatric behaviours has been attributed to both physical and psycho-social causes, yet no single school of thought has influenced our understanding of the growth and development of these behaviours above all others. Very often, the actual cause of the condition is of little relevance, either because the individual has been behaving this way for so long that he has forgotten how it all began, or because the behavioural problem is so acute that the major consideration is more one of life preserving interventions than analytical ones. Somehow the people responsible for the delivery of these interventions are aware of this and time is spent appropriate to the situation.

How do nurses prioritise so that they are able to function appropriately? The actual decision-making process will vary from person to person and institution to institution, but the dynamics are common to all. Information is communicated from the patient to the nurse. This nurse either communicates the information gathered to other nurses or carries out the next activity on her own. This involves tapping the body of knowledge available to nurses about human behaviour, disequilibrium, social interchange and need patterns. The nurse will then decide upon the best course of action, hopefully communicate this to others, including the patient, and carry that action out.

The key here is the word, 'communication'. What is common to both the behaviourists and the humanists, or those who work from a social or a medical perspective, is that the only real information that the nurse has about the patient is what she actually sees of him at the time of their meeting. This information is communicated by the patient. She also has second-hand information from records, comments of others and previous knowledge of the individual. This too has been communicated but via another medium, that of the written word. Finally, she also has comparative information in books, standard texts, previous cases and case studies, and that collective body of professional memories readily made available by her colleagues at a moment's notice. Only the first of these, the information communicated by the patient himself – and to some extent only that communicated at the point of contact as opposed to during previous meetings – can really provide an effective picture of what is happening to him, and is therefore the only accurate source of information. It would seem that what the nurse needs is not so much a philosophical basis on which to determine the cause of a behaviour but rather a communication device which enables her to make sense of it.

Part of the basic construct of the nursing process is its ability to act as a medium through which information can be passed from one source to another, or can be gathered, analysed and stored for future distribution. Thus, the nursing process's greatest single impact on the nursing profession has been its potential for increasing communication between patients and nurses, nurses and nurses, and nurses and other interested parties. The nursing process offers individual nurses a tool which can be used to tell them about their patients, and conversely tell the patient about the intentions of the nurse.

COMMUNICATION AND THE NURSING PROCESS

Communication is often divided into the spoken word and the unspoken, language and paralanguage, that which we tell each other by intention and that which we tell each other by default. We tend to choose the words we use to convey thoughts and feelings to each other, yet very often it is what we do not say that has more credence. For example, if a nurse is confronted by a patient who has been incontinent, and she says to the patient, 'That's OK. It could happen to anyone. Let's get sorted out', it sounds fine. But if as she says these words and the patient sees her pulling a face which seems to imply, 'This is awful', then the patient is likely to believe the nurse finds the situation distasteful. That is what the nurse has communicated to the patient, even if it is not the case. The consequent effect upon the patient, in what is already an embarrassing situation, is hardly likely to be that desired by quality nursing intervention. How can this situation be influenced by the use of the nursing process? and what is the link between the nursing process and non-verbal communication?

To better appreciate the answers to these two questions, we will first consider the influence that the nursing process has upon the verbal communication, firstly of nurses and then of patients.

NURSES' VERBAL COMMUNICATION

What is it that nurses communicate to their patients? Is there any standard format? Do they all say the same sort of things? The answer has to be a resounding no, but very often there are similarities in the nurses performance. The content of their communication falls into two groups:

- personal communication
- professional communication.

PERSONAL COMMUNICATION

Personal communication conveys information of a self-disclosing nature, about the nurse as a person. It serves the purpose of personal release for the nurse, and demonstrates to the patient the human qualities possessed by that nurse. It cannot be regulated, and some would argue that to do so would be to deny the humanisation process involved in nursing interaction. However, Peplau (1960) showed that nurses are often guilty of using this informal interactive process as a method of telling the patient to do something or to persuade him to go somewhere. In such cases, the communication process and the content are designed to benefit the nurse, and not the patient, so that the patient comes to believe that the nurse only comes to see him when she wants something from him. It does not matter that this might not have been the case, nor that there might be any number of reasons for believing otherwise, the fact is that this is the reality of the situation for the patient. If the nurse is unable to use personal communication as a means of humanising her interactions with patients, but uses it instead as a method by which to lull them into feeling that they are collaborating, then the sense of fellowship engendered by such activities is lost.

How much should the nurse involve herself in discussions where she herself is the topic of conversation? How much should the nurse try to use this form of disclosure as a method of distracting the patient from the pressures of his problems? Gibb & O'Brien (1990) found that nurses carrying out physical methods of care with the elderly often use a lighthearted and more jokey approach in their communications. However, they were at pains to point out that within a speech-act category list containing some 42 different types of communication process, jokes and general reassurance alone were not enough to make the patient feel confident and at ease. This is also likely to be the case with care designed to help with psychosocial problems.

The nursing process enables the nurse to monitor these informal discussions and, to a certain degree, it can also be used as a method of evaluating their performance. If the nurse designs care around a series of patient expressive objectives, then the actual speech content becomes the issue for the patient. This has to be documented in some way if the interactions between the nurse and the patient are to be of any value and if there is to be some progression through a relevant topic to some form of outcome. What the nurse says to the patient to prompt, stimulate or nudge the conversation around to the issues will need to be considered carefully if they are to be effective. This means that some of the apparently impromptu aspects of a patient–nurse conversation will have to be scripted beforehand. The danger is that this might reduce the apparent spontaneity of the conversation, and make the patient feel that he is being manipulated. Nonetheless, it enables the use of expressive objectives to take place within a therapeutic conversation that does not have all the pressure put upon the patient. If the nurse is also disclosing something, then the patient has the opportunity for reflection and circumspection.

The nursing process can also be used to evaluate the effectiveness of this communication process. If the objective for a patient is 'Jason will discuss why he always gets angry when his mother visits him', then there may be several ways that the nurse can begin the discussion. If she is too direct, then Jason is more than likely going to say the first thing that comes into his head. If the nurse is too indirect, then Jason may find he is controlling the conversation to the point where it serves no useful therapeutic purpose at all. However, if the nurse tries out certain opening gambits with the rest of the nursing team prior to beginning the conversation, then it will be she who directs the course of the conversation towards a more desirable conclusion. Jason is offered the opportunity of a discussion in which he can explore the reality of his own truth, rather than one constructed for him by the nurse. The actual openings or discussion areas can be written down, either in the progress notes or in the intervention section of the care plan. If they work, this should be documented. If they do not work, then the nurse must find out why and document this also so that others can learn from her mistake.

Types of introduction on a personal level might include:

- I always used to get upset when my mother came into my bedroom without knocking.
- I have been in such a rage with my parents that I refused to do anything when they were around.
- Sometimes my little girl will not let me in on a secret she has with one of her school friends, and it really drives me crazy.
- It really frightens me when I think of some of the things I have said to my mother and father over the years.

It can be seen that these introductory statements are geared towards are the nurse's objective for Jason. They are not about the same thing, but they are sufficiently related to be relevant, and they are not leading. If the nurse gets nowhere with any of them, then others will have to be tried, and if some record is kept as to what has been used beforehand nurses will not be guilty of using the same introductions over and over again until, eventually, they work because Jason gets so tired of resisting them.

PROFESSIONAL COMMUNICATION

Professional communication on a verbal level is either directed at the patient whilst in conversation with him, or it is on behalf of the patient in some form of case or clinical conference. It differs from personal communication in that it is directed specifically at either gathering or transmitting information about the clinical aspects of a patient. It focuses on the patient rather than the nurse, and it is designed to develop a greater understanding of the individual, his condition and the way that it affects the ability of that individual to deal with his own life. The information is used to construct an action plan for that individual, either as a care strategy or for discharge, admission or re-admission.

As might be expected from this form of communication, it often use professional jargon, and as such it excludes those who have not had medical or nurse education. Professional communication uses codes – consisting of such things as diagnoses, clinical terms, medications and methods of care – in such a way as to enable those who use it to short-circuit the normal processes of explanation and conformation. Hence communication is speeded up and, in theory, more work can be done. The reality of such methods of communication is, however, that many of the specific and individual aspects of a patient's presentation and performance are reduced to generalities such as 'auditory hallucinations', or 'disorientation'. To enable the professional to be more specific, they have to introduce more descriptive speech content once again. This may be regarded as diluting the 'professional' nature of the communication; the fact that it might be more effective seems not to be considered.

Fisher and Todd (1986) explored various forms of professional communication patterns within different institutional settings, and discovered that the consumer – in this case the patient – was often excluded from conversations held about them by the professional because the professional used speech codes that the consumer could not understand. This of course is one of the functions of professional languages. Goffman (1961) also noted that the language used by the professionals excluded patients, and he saw this as a method of controlling them. Thirty years later, researchers still report similar activities taking place (Lanceley 1985, Topf 1988, Scott 1990). To some extent such linguistic practice amongst nurses reflects the approach adopted by other medical and paramedical agencies (Stein 1985, Coleman & Burton 1985), but when balanced against the needs of the patient it can only be seen as counterproductive.

It is the patients who suffer when nurses use language that outsiders cannot fully comprehend. This may happen on two levels:

- *Level 1.* When the nurse uses language within the confines of a straightforward patient–nurse conversation which is too technical for the patient to understand, and which the nurse fails to explain. The patient, not wishing to seem uneducated, or rude, simply nods his head, and the nurse carries on totally oblivious to the problems being generated.

- *Level 2*. This is when the nurse approximates or 'rounds down' patient behaviour to the recognised type that most closely resembles it, because there is not a technical expression which fully or accurately describes the observed behaviour. This has knock-on effects. The nurses who receive this information about the patient do their own 'rounding down' until the exact nature of the patient's behaviour has been totally lost. Such a misuse of professional communication is called 'discommunication'.

Gray (1989) feels that such game playing is the result of nurses attempting to manipulate situations as a tactic to cope with the pressures of work. This may be the case. However, whatever the reason, the result is that the patient is disadvantaged and therefore cannot make full use of the clinical resources that should be available to him. Gray feels that one solution is to teach communication skills and awareness within a staff development programme. However, another, and more immediate arena in which to tackle such difficulties is the workplace itself, and within that workplace the medium through which nursing interventions are constructed and delivered – the nursing process.

How can the nursing process contribute to a more effective use of professional communication? In fact, the question is more about the communication content than the communication itself. Whenever two people meet they automatically communicate with each other, but it is the nature of what is said that can be influenced, in this case, by the use of the nursing process.

Level 1

How do you combat a situation where nurses use language in open conversation which the patient cannot understand? Why not simply say to the nurse concerned 'Be careful what you say'. The

answer is simple, it does not work. Things have to be far more controlled if they are to be effective.

Firstly, nurses involved in analytical or insightful work with patients should see as part of their role the necessity to build into the care plan a component which increases the patient's knowledge and understanding of his own condition and the methods of coming to terms with it. This means using the language of the professional. Why? Because other professionals are just as likely to slip into this communication shorthand as nurses, so that the patient has a fair chance of understanding what is being said and it increases the quality of the interaction. Of course, an even greater spin-off is the increase in the patient's confidence and self-esteem derived from his increased ability to understand. He too feels that he belongs to this group of people that appear to know what they are about. Nurses should not underestimate their influence upon their patients.

The process of recording this information should take place either on the care plan itself in the sections outlining intervention and evaluation, or in some complementary record such as progress notes. The more that the nurse is encouraged to use the intervention as a method of increasing the patient's understanding and awareness, the more successful the patient is likely to be. Words, phrases and titles should be selected that are appropriate to the patient's current care programme. They should appear on the care plan in a sequential fashion and, once they have been explained carefully, and in context, to the patient, nurses should be encouraged to use them regularly whilst talking to that patient.

Also on the care plan, though perhaps as an evaluative statement, should appear a warning to nurses to look out for facial expressions from the patient which denote that discommunication may be taking place. Once the nurse has begun to formalise this process, the interactive activities between selected patients and nurses become more meaningful and effective. Without such vigilance, other, less professional, explanations may start to creep into the nurses communication activities. The process of looking out for confusion and actually telling the patient what is meant produces a more competent relationship that has the potential for a more therapeutic result. The nursing process itself cannot influence the communication but, because of the continuity and regularity that it promotes, it can act as the medium through which greater understanding takes place.

Level 2

How can the nursing process influence the way that a nurse uses professional communication with other professionals? Surely nurses need to be seen to be on equal terms with other professionals, and the language they use is the best way to do this?

The truth is that the more effective you are as a practitioner the more you are accepted as an equal. Trying to copy, and doing it badly, may be a sign of flattery but it is a sign of weakness. Nurses certainly do not have to copy others to assert their claim to professionalism or, for that matter, competency.

ROLES AND PROFESSIONAL COMMUNICATION

The professional language used by medical staff reflects what they do, which in psychiatry is often diagnostic and prescriptive. Nurses may also be diagnostic, but not in the medical sense. Nurses are trying to convey the effects of the patient's condition upon his ability to lead some sort of independent existence. It should be obvious that nurses should be using their professional communications to reflect this. In other words their speech content should be descriptive, conveying what they see, hear, etc. The nursing process can influence professional communication in one specific way: by demanding that nurses always use this descriptive form of communication when they write information down on the care plans, and on all the other auxiliary documentation associated with them. This serves two purposes.

1. It ensures that nurses do not become tempted to use language which does not reflect their clinical role.

2. It ensures that nurses use language which reflects their patients' behaviour.

Hence, statements such as 'Has oscillations of his emotional equilibrium' are written as, 'Sometimes he seems to be happy and at other times less so'. Or, 'Some evidence of first rank Schniderian symptomatology exists' becomes 'He thinks he can hear a voice talking about him to someone else'. The symptomatic codes are not necessary for the delivery of nursing care, and they certainly would not help the patient to understand his condition any better. They may be very damaging in that the patient may consider doing nothing about his situation simply because it has been legitimised by a medical diagnosis.

If nursing team members were regularly audited by their colleagues to ensure that statements written within the nursing process were accurate and effective in descriptive terms, this would go a long way towards the development of consistent nursing communication. Students of nursing, exposed to this form of clinical talk from the beginning of their courses, would be less likely to use other less appropriate types of language, and gradually nurses would feel more confident about what they both wrote and said within the confines of the multi-disciplinary team.

It is perhaps worth considering why so many nurses, and in particular students of nursing, feel so obliged to use the more medically oriented form of professional language. It is probably a complex combination of all sorts of psychosocial factors, but at the heart of it is the sense of belonging that one gets from using a special language among a group of people who use that same special language. It is almost as if nurses wanted to be doctors. But no, nurses do not want to be doctors or, in this case, psychiatrists; but they do feel the need to compete with them for seniority within the clinical arena. This may sound strange but such competition is not restricted to nursing and medicine, it happens in any environment where more than one group of people have some say in what takes place. However, the effects in nursing are that nurses become reluctant to contradict doctors and make decisions about care for which they should have the ultimate responsibility. Doctors and nurses in psychiatry have to work in a complementary fashion if they are to provide quality care for their patients. Nurses should not feel that doctors should tell them how to nurse.

The other effect of nurses' sense of powerlessness is that in stating what appears to be the obvious whilst in conversation with others they may feel that their part within the clinical whole is seen as less important. However, nurses writing on care plans have to do so in such a way that others know exactly what is happening, otherwise care cannot be delivered as it was agreed and intended. Why then is there any need to change this when talking to others? Nurses are far more effective as team members when they use the nursing process to demonstrate the rationale for their input into the care programme. This means that they speak the words of the patient within the decision-making arena known as the multi-disciplinary team. In this way, they are more likely to get for the patient, just what the patient might want for himself.

VERBAL COMMUNICATION AND PATIENT/NURSE EQUALITY

In 1960, Hilgard Peplau was already exploring the interactive activities of patients and nurses in psychiatric settings from a sociological point of view. Part of her work considered the effects of the then relatively new process of nursing on the communication patterns being used. It is interesting to consider what she said, over 30 years ago, about a situation which still exists within developing care delivery systems. She looked at what was actually said, and the way the information was presented, when nursing staff were involved in dynamic clinical activity, i.e. when actions and strategies were being thought out carefully before being put into practice. She observed that the nurse's 'social chit-chat' was replaced by a more effective interchange which she described as a 'more responsible use of words' (Peplau 1960). She felt that this made an important contribution to increasing the patient's understanding of what was happening to him, and of what he might require of the care environment. More significantly, Peplau felt that patient–nurse conversations were far more meaningful when nurses took more responsibility for their part in the verbal interchange.

This shift in emphasis, from having conversations with patients which have little or no effect upon the therapeutic context of the clinical environment to those which demand a higher level of patient participation, coincided with the development of the nursing process, and the latter's influence cannot be denied. Contained within the basic philosophy of the nursing process is a belief in the basic equality of all those involved in the development of care, including the recipient. A basic conversation between equals contains a sharing and an honesty which enables both parties to say what they feel without fear of retribution, with neither being disadvantaged by the other. Equality is expressed within a conversation when one individual gives information to another so that they both know as much as each other. Equality is expressed by one individual letting the other have his or her say. Equality allows people to have different points of view, without falling out over them. Above all else, equality in a conversation means that each participant is able to enjoy his or her own expression of the truth of a matter.

This connection between the action of equal speaking and the underlying approach through which it may be facilitated, in this case the nursing process, is not restricted to care environments alone; but whether it be found in a car production plant, a football team, a higher educational establishment or a large department store, it has certain features which need to be considered.

1. What individuals say to each other is often pre-arranged or carefully thought out.
2. Each participant allows the other to say what he or she thinks.
3. In formal environments, a record is kept as to what has been said.
4. Each conversation serves a purpose.
5. One individual does not use his or her knowledge to influence or control the other, especially if he or she does not have access to that same knowledge.

6. The participants feel that they are on equal terms.
7. No games playing is endulged in.
8. The more the participants talk to each other the more they know about each other and about the individual worlds that they represent.
9. The participants do not take advantage of each other.
10. The participants do not interrupt each other.

It could perhaps be argued that any one of these points are representative of an effective use of the nursing process. The nursing process cannot be used properly if the nurse feels the necessity to control the patient, the care or the total situation. The nurse cannot be effective if the patient feels that he will be punished in some way if he does not do that he is told. If the nurse tries to manipulate the patient into doing things he does not want to do then he will respond in the same way as any other hurt or offended person. Professional conversations between patients and nurses need to be planned and organised if they are to achieve a particular goal. Success needs to be worked at. It does not just happen. There has to be a reason for it. Nurses need to work with their patients to find out the cause-and-effect connections, and this demands that their conversations contain clearly defined objectives.

CARE STATEMENTS

If the components of an equal interchange between two individuals appear to have the same characteristics as those associated with the use of an effective nursing process, could it be possible that the connections work in reverse? In other words, if the nursing process is working well, will this affect the conversations that are held between the patient and the nurse? The chances are that the two are interactive and interdependent to such a degree that it is not possible to separate them in this way. If the nursing process cannot work without the element of equality being present, then it follows that the conversations being held by the patient and the nurse are already exhibiting those same qualities.

The statements made by the nurses within their documentation and on behalf of their patients are also likely to reflect this element of equality. Similarly, the style and nature of the interventions chosen by patients and nurses will give another indication of the equality that exists between them. For example, the use of expressive objectives reflects the nurse's willingness to allow the patient to have his own say in what is happening to him. Nurses who continually use behavioural objectives, even for emotional and intellectual difficulties, are usually attempting to manipulate either the patient or his environment in some way (Sturmey 1988). Expressive, or experiential objectives allow the patient to say and do what is real for him, although this may conflict with what the nurse believes. As we have already seen, this is permissible in a relationship based upon equality. Intervention activities which allow the patient the same freedom will also reflect this tolerance. Examples of this include cognitive psychotherapeutic activities or, on a less formal level, the use of validation therapy with the elderly mentally ill (Bleathman 1988).

This last example may be used to illustrate the difference between prescriptive (and consequently controlling) activities and evocative (and subsequently more patient-oriented) activities. Consider first a prescriptive technique for contending with the problems related to a patient's inability to interpret correctly what is going on around them. This is commonly called disorientation, but does not tell you about the condition. The patient makes the wrong sense of in-coming sensory information and, as a consequence, everything that transpires is likely to conflict with the patient's own beliefs and may cause uncertainty and alarm. The nurse elects to use some form of orientation therapy. Information is written on a board or chart and displayed in a prominent part of the ward for all the patients to see. Signposts are placed at strategic points indicating key places on the ward, such as toilets, bedrooms, etc. The patient has to refer to these reference points, so that if he goes to the wrong bedroom or gets the wrong time and place he is regarded as being in the wrong. In effect, he has failed. If this form of therapy is not supported by some other approach, then it has proven only one thing, that the nurse is more able to remember than the patient. It has achieved nothing for the patient.

Consider now the effects of choosing validation therapy to complement the orientation activity. Validation therapy is a method of communicating with people who are disoriented. It uses specific interactive techniques (which it would be out of place to describe here) the effect of which is to allow the patient to create his own truth and to generate self-worth in individuals who would otherwise be more likely to experience uncertainty. The therapy works particularly well with expressive objectives, because they use the same approach to patient's beliefs and feelings. The use of validation therapy shows that the nurse wants the patient to explore things for himself and that she will allow him to develop his own understanding of what is happening. The patient cannot be wrong; he is equal, not inferior, to the nurse. There is no competition between them. The nurse has chosen to use a form of therapy which allows the patient to be himself, even though he may not be able to tell who everyone else is.

Is this choice of therapy indicative of effective nursing process? Or is the desire to indulge in communication which reflects equality between the patient and the nurse more a matter of intuition? Certainly, the nurse has got to feel that she is equal to the patient to have any chance of bringing it about. However, even if the choice is intuitive, making it work as an effective medium through which therapeutic actions may take place is something that has to be worked at and rehearsed time and time again. It cannot be expressed except through the sense of caring and, as will be seen, often it is the non-verbal communication which reinforces it.

The nursing process is not about forms and documentation, though of course these are important if it is to be shared with others. No, the nursing process is something which reflects the individual nurse's personal philosophy towards her patients. If the nurse believes that she and her patients are equal then the nursing process becomes something that you 'do', not something that you have to work at. Certainly,

all the auxiliary actions described in this book have to be practised, but they in turn are the tricks of the nursing process, they are not the nursing process itself. It is something that nurses feel, it is expressed through a sense of caring and uses verbal communication as the tool by which it is put into practice. It follows, therefore, that if nurses use effective problem-oriented and 'equal' communication, the nursing process, if not already being used, is certainly not far away.

NURSES' NON-VERBAL COMMUNICATION

Nurses' non-verbal communication, or paralanguage, has the same purpose as verbal communication in that it tells the patient about the nurse. However, it cannot be considered in the same way as verbal communication – i.e. as either professional or personal – because it just happens. Some of it might, however, be regarded in a negative way as being unprofessional.

NEGATIVE USE OF NON-VERBAL LANGUAGE

Unlike verbal communication, the nurse often cannot control what she conveys to her patients on a non-verbal level. For example, the nurse may say verbally to the patient, 'Between us we will construct your care so that it best suits your needs'. This short message conveys to the patient that they are going to work together, that they are going to make something, that it is going to be the best it can be and that it is especially designed for the patient. Very professional and very sound. However, the nurse was out late last night. She is tired and it has been a difficult and taxing shift. She is ready to go home. As she turns to leave the patient she lets out a small sigh. It might mean nothing and she was not even aware that she did it, but the patient heard it. Did it convey to him that the nurse had been out late last night and had worked a difficult shift? That she was feeling satisfied at the work she was doing but, like any other worker getting to the end of a day's work, was looking forward to going home? No, to the patient it probably said, 'Gosh, you are boring and I did not really mean anything I just said. If we do produce this care it will be in my time and only because I cannot find anyone else to do it'. Or if it did not convey quite this message, certainly something similar.

The nurse had no intention of betraying the fact that she was tired because she knew that the patient might construe this as being in some way related to him. She would not have transmitted such a message because it would have been counterproductive and might have damaged the relationship built up between them. Yet she did it anyway. Why? Because she was tired? Because she really did not care? Because she was trying to say something to the patient? Who knows, and in any case it does not really matter why it happened, just that it did.

Of course, paralanguage can be a gesture, a movement, different intensity of eye contact or lack of it, facial expressions, posture, tone of voice, even the repeated failure to remember someone's name. Always turning up late to an agreed patient meeting, or wearing too much make-up and looking over-dressed can also be regarded as non-verbal cues. When used effectively, verbal cues can convey warmth, truth, honesty and compassion, yet they also have a negative aspect when they convey a sense of indifference or even hostility.

POSITIVE USE OF NON-VERBAL LANGUAGE

Consider a positive use of non-verbal communication. A patient is feeling particularly low and sad. She has little knowledge of what she wants out of life and is lonely and dejected. In her mind she is worth very little, and she cannot for the life of her see any reason why anyone should be the least bit interested in her. Her nurse, an efficient young man, walks through the room. He stops and appears to be looking around for something. Whilst she is watching he turns in her direction, smiles and raises his hand in acknowledgement. She suddenly realises that he was looking straight at her. Before she can do anything in reply he has moved on again. This

happens several times during the morning. Each time, he seems to be seeking her out especially, and he always smiles. At lunchtime he comes over to her and talks to her about several things. She is quite pleased that he does. She feels that he cares. Why? Because even when he apparently had nothing to say to her he was still concerned about her.

NON-VERBAL COMMUNICATION AND THE NURSING PROCESS

How can the nursing process be used to aid the use of non-verbal communication. In truth, the possibilities are limited. As we have already seen, unlike the verbal type, non-verbal communication has a tendency to happen without being scripted. Yet this does not always have to be the case. The strength of non-verbal communication lies in the fact that people are often totally unaware of non-verbal communication cues, they simply respond to them. This can be used both as a social tool and as a therapeutic strategy. Look again at the positive example of paralanguage given above. What the patient did not realise was that on the care plan the nurse had written that the patient was to be acknowledged openly every hour, no matter what she was doing. The nurse simply carried out this activity with a little exaggeration to enhance the effect. As we have seen, this effect was to give the patient the sensation of being cared about, without any words ever being used.

Of course, if the patient had collaborated in the development of the care plan she would have seen this statement written and the whole activity would have been wasted. However, the actual nature of this approach would not necessarily have to be explained fully. Also, it is the action which is important here, not the words, and written words come into this category just the same as spoken ones. Hence, even if the patient had been fully aware of the entry on the care plan, the action of acknowledgement without any accompanying verbal action would have been powerful enough to signify that the deed itself was important to the nurse. By his actions, the nurse communicated that the patient was important. In fact words at this time may well have diluted the effect of the action. What it enabled the nurse to do was to go to the patient later to discuss important things with her without her feeling that he was only interested in her when he wanted her for something, Peplau's famous conclusion once again (1960).

One may ask, 'Why bother writing this, or any other non-verbal communication, down on paper at all? Why not just do it?' The answer is, for the same reason that much of the nursing process actions need to be documented, so that people can use the care plans as a point of operational reference. Very few nurses are able to remember all the things they have to do in their working day without some reference to a diary or plan. The care plan acts to remind the nurse of the things to be done. Some wards or teams have shift planners which serve the same purpose. These are time-gridded sheets of paper, and the nurse extracts the necessary actions for the shift from the care plan and transfers it to the shift planner in the appropriate time slot. Hence, something which had to be carried out every hour, such as acknowledging a specific patient, would appear seven or eight times on the planner, next to the time it had to be carried out. Other items that needed less input might appear only once or twice, but always next to the appropriate time. All the nurse needs to do is refer to the planner every once and a while to see what should happen next. At the end of the shift, the planner would be torn up and destroyed, and a new one made out by the nurse during the next day's handover.

In this case, the recognition of the patient on an apparently intuitive level might well have been carefully scripted, just like good professional verbal communication, and recorded on the shift planner to happen once an hour, followed by a half-an-hour of more exploratory discussion. The one approach, in this case, complements the other.

Any form of non-verbal communication could be scripted in to reinforce the actions and verbal exchanges of the nurse. At first sight, this might appear to be game playing, contradicting what was said earlier about honesty within an 'equal' conversation. However, it is not game playing and it certainly does not compromise equality within the interactions. This is because all the nurse is doing is taking the trouble to convert a normally unconscious activity into a conscious one. Taking the trouble to select the correct and complementary approach or action, writing it down and carrying it out to good effect are all professional actions designed to enhance the patient's sensation of reassurance. If anything, such actions demonstrate equality rather than the opposite, because they show that the nurse cares enough about the patient to do the job properly.

CONCLUSION

Throughout this book, we have seen that communication is the medium through which the nursing process is expressed. This chapter has tried to explore the nature of verbal and non-verbal communication when used to best effect within the nursing process. The nursing process demands that the nurse develops an awareness of herself within the care scenario, if actions, strategies and interventions are to have the necessary impact upon the patient. Very often, statements written on the care plans or other ancillary documents are messages for the nurse to remind her of the need to do things the right way, or to take time to do them in a certain way. In this case, she is simply communicating with herself, keeping herself informed, in touch and enlightened.

Communication can be either formal or informal, professional or personal, verbal or non-verbal, but it is always important. Use of the nursing process implies a recognition of equality between the patient and the nurse, and this in turn is put into practice through the use of 'equal' patient–nurse communication.

Finally, it should be said that not all nurses possess the ability to communicate on either a verbal or non-verbal level with their patients and generate this sense of equality. Those that are able to do so will undoubtedly find it easier to carry out the nursing process than those who cannot, for this belief that patients and nurses are of equal status lies at the heart of the nursing process. The tricks of the nursing process, the forms, the documents, writing down objectives and working out time scales, can be taught to any nurse, but the nursing process itself, as a working philosophy, is something that cannot be taught; it has to be believed, and believed in.

REFERENCES

Bleathman C 1988 Validation therapy with the demented elderly. Journal of Advanced Nursing 13: 511–514

Coleman H, Burton J 1985 Aspects of control in the dentist–patient relationship. International Journal of the Sociology of Language. Language and Work 2: The health professions 51: 75–104

Fisher S, Todd A D (eds) 1986 Communication in institutional contexts: social interaction and social structure. In: Discourses and institutional authority: medicine, education and law, Vol XIX. Ablex Publishing Corporation, Norwood, New Jersey

Gibb H, O'Brien B 1990 Jokes and reassurance are not enough: ways in which nurses relate through conversation with elderly clients. Journal of Advanced Nursing 15: 1389–1401

Goffman E 1961 Asylums–essays on the social situation of mental patients and other inmates. Pelican, Middlesex

Gray J 1989 Communication skills. Chpt.6 In: Dodwell H, Lathlean J (eds) Management and professional development for nurses. Harper & Row, London

Lanceley A 1985 Use of controlling language in the rehabilitation of the elderly. Journal of Advanced Nursing 10: 125–135

Peplau H 1960 Talking with patients. American Journal of Nursing 60: 964–966

Scott M 1990 Language as a quality issue. Senior Nurse 10(7): 26–27

Stein H F 1985 The psycho-dynamics of medical practice. University of California Press, Los Angeles

Sturmey P 1988 Writing behavioural objectives: an evaluation of a simple, inexpensive method. Journal of Advanced Nursing 13: 496–500

Topf M 1988 Verbal interpersonal responses. Journal of Psychosocial Nursing 26(7): 8–16

SUGGESTED READING

Burnard P 1990 Learning to care for the spirit. Nursing Standard 4(18): 38–39

Kitson A 1987 A comparative analysis of lay-caring and professional (nursing) caring relationships. International Journal of Nursing Studies 24(2): 155–165

Salvage J 1990 The theory and practice of the 'new nursing'. Nursing Times (occasional papers) 86(4): 42–45

Index